Psychotherapy and Apha

Psychotherapy and Aphasia: Interventions for Emotional Wellbeing and Relationships is an exciting international collaboration among clinical neuropsychologists, speech and language therapists and family therapists that details a range of innovative psychotherapeutic interventions to enable people with communication disorders and their families to access meaningful support.

People with aphasia and other acquired communication disorders can face significant challenges accessing emotional support. Many traditional forms of psychotherapy are based on spoken language, rendering it inaccessible for many people with communication disorders. But the book details a range of techniques that move away from reliance on spoken language, including total communication strategies, the use of meaningful objects, experiential process, group experience and mind-body practices.

Featuring clinical examples which cover a range of stroke and neurology service contexts, the book includes contributions from a range of therapeutic models; from speech and language therapy and family therapy to clinical neuropsychology, cognitive-behavioural, systemic, narrative and mind-body traditions. It therefore provides clinicians with a wide-range of practical and theoretical tools to explore when supporting survivors who experience psychological distress during rehabilitation. It is the only book aimed at both speech and language therapists and psychotherapists, and will open up new pathways to support.

Kate H. Meredith worked as a speech and language therapist in acquired brain injury and neurology services for 15 years, retraining as a family and systemic psychotherapist to support families with the relational impact of communication disorders. Kate currently works in child and adolescent mental health services and independently in Cardiff.

Dr Giles N. Yeates is Editor of the journal and book series *Neuro-Disability & Psychotherapy*, in addition to the Brain Injury book series (Routledge). As a clinical neuropsychologist in community neuro-rehabilitation, his clinical work and research focus on the innovation of psychological therapies and support of relationships following acquired brain injury. Dr Yeates is currently innovating the use of Tai Ji in neuro-rehabilitation.

Neuro-Disability & Psychotherapy: Specialist Topics

Series Editor: Dr Giles N. Yeates

Originally the *Neuro-Disability & Psychotherapy* journal, this book series covers themed topics around psychotherapy for a range of neurological disorders.

Previous titles in the series:

Volume One
Eastern Influences on Neuropsychotherapy
Accepting, Soothing, and Stilling Cluttered and Critical Minds, 1st Edition
Edited by Giles N. Yeates and Gavin Farrell

Volume Two
Psychotherapy and Aphasia
Interventions for Emotional Wellbeing and Relationships
Edited by Kate H. Meredith and Giles N. Yeates

For further information about this series please visit: www.routledge.com/psychology/series/KARNNDP

Psychotherapy and Aphasia

Interventions for Emotional Wellbeing and Relationships

Volume Two of the *Neuro-Disability & Psychotherapy: Specialist Topics* Series

Edited by Kate H. Meredith and Giles N. Yeates

Routledge
Taylor & Francis Group
LONDON AND NEW YORK

First published 2020
by Routledge
2 Park Square, Milton Park, Abingdon, Oxon OX14 4RN

and by Routledge
52 Vanderbilt Avenue, New York, NY 10017

Routledge is an imprint of the Taylor & Francis Group, an informa business

British Library Cataloguing-in-Publication Data
A catalogue record for this book is available from the British Library

Library of Congress Cataloging-in-Publication Data
A catalog record for this book has been requested

ISBN: 9780367141394 (hbk)
ISBN: 9780367141400 (pbk)
ISBN: 9780429030482 (ebk)

Typeset in Times New Roman
by Apex CoVantage, LLC

MIX
Paper from responsible sources
FSC™ C013985
FSC www.fsc.org

Printed in the United Kingdom
by Henry Ling Limited

Contents

Editors' foreword vii
KATE H. MEREDITH, GILES N. YEATES

1 **Time to step up: a call for the speech pathology profession to utilise stepped psychological care for people with aphasia post stroke** 1
BROOKE RYAN, LINDA WORRALL, JASVINDER SEKHON, CAROLINE BAKER, MARCELLA CARRAGHER, JAYCIE BOHAN, EMMA POWER, MIRANDA ROSE, NINA SIMMONS-MACKIE, LEANNE TOGHER, IAN KNEEBONE

2 **The importance of syntax in making meaning and emotional adjustment: a brief psychodynamically oriented intervention in receptive aphasia** 17
AONGHUS RYAN

3 **A personal construct psychology approach to aphasia** 33
CATHY SPARKES

4 **Supporting families with aphasia to explore relationships** 53
KATE H. MEREDITH

5 **A preliminary study of "Laboratorio di Conversazione Narrativa": group psychotherapy supporting communication for people with aphasia** 80
STEFANO MONTE, MARISTELLA CRIELESI, MARCELLA DI PIETRO, MARIATERESA MATERA, KATE H. MEREDITH, ROSSELLA MUÒ

6 **Structured narrative therapy for children with acquired brain injury and severe communication difficulties** **95**
ALISON PERKINS

7 **Mindfulness interventions for people with aphasia – case evidence from individual and group therapy formats** **107**
MARISTELLA CRIELESI, LAUREN ROCHE, GIULIA MONOPOLI, GILES N. YEATES, STEFANO MONTE

8 **The potential contribution of mind-body interventions within psychological support following aphasia: a conceptual review and case study** **136**
GILES N. YEATES

Index 165

Editors' foreword

Kate H. Meredith and Giles N. Yeates

Since Freud, the professional provision of emotional support has been historically defined as the "talking cure" and is delivered through, and heavily dependent on, language. Aphasia and related communication disorders in neurological conditions challenge conventionally held ideas and assumptions relating to psychotherapy, emotional support in a broader sense, and the interconnection of language and relationships. These challenges are sadly often not met at the level of service provision, with the result being that survivors of stroke and other neurological conditions who experience psychological distress and isolation are then denied access to meaningful forms of support. Their exclusion from the talking cure is particularly cruel, as the effort to access help to manage distress caused by communication difficulties becomes yet a further instance of disability, restriction and social exclusion from significant others and potential resources within society.

Thankfully, clinicians and researchers have noticed the cruelty and unfair discrimination of this situation, and efforts have been made to both think outside of the box in developing forms of emotional support, and to systematically address inequalities in structural exclusions within service pathways. Over the same period, the broader psychotherapy field has seen an unprecedented burgeoning of diverse forms of emotional support, broadening to encompass approaches that are founded as much on visual sense-making resources as verbal, focused on relationships as opposed to an isolated individual to talk to in a consulting room, and focused more on the body than talking in a disembodied, linguistic-heavy encounter.

This volume of collected papers on the topic of psychotherapy following aphasia thankfully represents the fruits of all of these contemporary developments, arriving at a range of diverse approaches, ideas and techniques that should equip readers with a diverse toolbox in their work. The second volume in the *Neuro-Disability & Psychotherapy: Specialist Topics* series, the contributions herein from leading experts and pioneers in their field should empower clinicians to move towards people with aphasia and their significant others, and to start a meaningful exchange of shared meaning and support, rather than turn away in a state of hopelessness and disempowerment (for both service users and clinicians). While the range of orientations represented here (cognitive-behavioural, personal construct, neuropsychoanalytical, systemic, narrative, mindfulness and mind-body traditions) may each appeal to different readers, we hope it is this diversity of ideas and forms of practice that overcomes the historical inertia associated with the professional provision of emotional support for people with aphasia. Furthermore, this project has emerged between the two core professions, speech and language therapy (as termed in the UK) and clinical neuropsychology, and the results are bigger than the sum of the two professional halves – neither profession could have yielded such diversity across chapters in isolation.

We would like this collaboration to be a point of inspiration for multi-disciplinary/inter-disciplinary teams in neurological services around the world and encourage similar cross-professional dialogue. We hope this will lead to the development of innovative opportunities that will equip people with aphasia to make sense of and manage distress secondary to communication difficulties, and feel less alone.

Kate H. Meredith, Guest Co-Editor, Speech and Language Therapist & Family and Systemic Psychotherapist
Giles N. Yeates, Editor, Clinical Neuropsychologist, Couples Therapist and Tai Ji Instructor

Chapter 1

Time to step up

A call for the speech pathology[1] profession to utilise stepped psychological care for people with aphasia post stroke

Brooke Ryan[2,7], Linda Worrall[2,7], Jasvinder Sekhon[3,7], Caroline Baker[3,7], Marcella Carragher[3,7], Jaycie Bohan[2], Emma Power[4,7], Miranda Rose[3,7], Nina Simmons-Mackie[5], Leanne Togher[4,7], Ian Kneebone[6,7]

Introduction

Stroke often results in significant psychological upheaval and strain (Brumfitt, 1993; Gainotti, 1997; LaFond, 1993; Lincoln, Kneebone, Macniven, & Morris, 2012; Lincoln & Kneebone, 2012; Robinson, 2010; Tanner, 2003; Thomas & Lincoln, 2006). Lincoln and Kneebone (2012) report on the prevalence and variety of psychological conditions after stroke, including depression (30%), involuntary emotional expression disorder (20%-30%), post-traumatic stress reaction (27%), apathy (22%-28%), generalised anxiety disorder (10%-30%), catastrophic reaction (20%), fear of falling (60%), and anger (17%-35%). The prevalence of psychological conditions among people with stroke is likely to continue to increase alongside Australia's increasing ageing population and accompanied increased incidence of stroke. More than 420,000 Australian stroke survivors currently live in the community, and this is set to increase to approximately 700,000 by 2032 (Deloitte Access Economics, 2013).

Concurrent with these distressing psychological outcomes, a stroke may result in a range of physical and communication sequelae. One of the most common communication difficulties is aphasia, which is a language impairment that can affect reading, writing, talking and understanding and limits everyday conversations (Hallowell & Chapey, 2008). Approximately 30 per cent of stroke survivors have aphasia, and, whilst substantial language recovery is possible, many people will live with aphasia for the rest of their lives (Flowers et al., 2016). Aphasia appears to be a risk factor for poor mental health (Kutlubaev & Hackett, 2014; Menlove et al., 2015). Up to 70 per cent of individuals with stroke and aphasia have depression (Kauhanen et al., 2000), and up to 44 per cent have anxiety (Morris, Eccles, Ryan, & Kneebone, 2017). People with post-stroke aphasia also often report other psychological impacts, including changes in identity and sense of self, feelings of frustration and/or isolation, negative self-esteem, reduced coping abilities, stress, distress, reduced optimism and hope, changed life satisfaction and wellbeing (Brumfitt, 2006; Cruice, Hill, Worrall, & Hickson, 2010; Hilari, Needle, & Harrison, 2012; Parr, 2001; Shadden, Hagstrom, & Koski, 2008).

The communication disability imposed by aphasia influences psychological wellbeing and restricts participation in activities of choice (Cruice, Worrall, Hickson, & Murison, 2003; Hackett, Anderson, House, & Halteh, 2008; Hilari & Byng, 2009; Hilari, Wiggins, Roy, Byng, & Smith, 2003). This has a spiralling effect, with resultant poor psychological wellbeing in turn reducing frequency and enjoyment of activities and participation in previously enjoyed life roles, and interfering with adjustment and participation in rehabilitation (Brown, Worrall, Davidson, & Howe, 2010; Carota, Staub, & Bogousslavsky, 2002; Code & Herrmann, 2003; Cruice, Worrall, & Hickson, 2011; Fucetola et al., 2006). It is not surprising that one recent study found that in the first 12 months post stroke, low mood was consistently and negatively associated with successfully living with aphasia (Worrall, Hudson, Khan, Ryan, & Simmons-Mackie, 2017). Another reason why this population is particularly at risk of poor mental health is that aphasia after stroke is associated with greater disability, increased reliance on rehabilitation services and increased likelihood of being discharged to a care setting rather than home from hospital (Flowers et al., 2016).

There is a significant gap between clinical need and service provision to support psychological health in people with aphasia. The Stroke Foundation in Australia has consistently identified that access to mental health services post stroke is extremely limited (Stroke Foundation, 2018). Their latest audit found that 50% of patients had some degree of mood impairment post stroke yet one third of services reported no access to clinical or neuropsychologists in stroke rehabilitation (Stroke Foundation, 2018). These figures relate to the general stroke population, and therefore the level of psychological services provided to people with aphasia are likely to be much lower given the challenges of psychological service provision to individuals with communication disability (Ryan, Bohan, & Kneebone, 2019). People with aphasia are therefore vulnerable to poor mental health that will likely deteriorate over time because of insufficient access to treatment and support.

Mental health studies typically exclude people with aphasia because the research procedures, outcome measures or treatments are determined to be inaccessible to them (Campbell, Skidmore, Whyte, & Matthews, 2015; Townend, Brady, & McLaughlan, 2007). The impact of this exclusion perpetuates the disparity in stroke care for people with aphasia. Brady, Fredrick, and Williams (2013) described this phenomenon as "an unacceptable stroke-specific variation of the 'inverse care law' where people with the highest needs have the poorest evidence base and receive the least research attention" (p. 193). This lack of evidence in mental health research may also promote the false notion that people with aphasia cannot engage in any kind of psychotherapeutic or mental health–focussed intervention, largely on account of communication barriers (Dalemans, Wade, van den Heuvel, & de Witte, 2009).

Speech pathologists may be well placed to facilitate access to mental health services in people with aphasia after stroke. They have expertise in providing communication support and have a comprehensive understanding of the pervasive impact of aphasia. Speech pathologists often take on the role of "communication broker" between a person with aphasia and the stroke team. Unfortunately, a lack of formal psychological therapy training means speech pathologists may feel either limited in terms of scope of practice to deliver mental health supports/interventions or under-skilled to do so (Sekhon, Douglas, & Rose, 2015). Approximately 45 per cent of speech pathologists do not formally screen for mental health issues in their patients with aphasia and two thirds do not address wellbeing as part of their management (Sekhon et al., 2015). Whilst some people with stroke do have access to mental health practitioners, these practitioners often do not have the necessary skills to serve this group (Northcott, Simpson, Moss, Ahmed, & Hilari, 2016).

The answer to the limited psychological training speech pathologists receive may seem obvious: that speech pathologists train mental health practitioners to work with people with aphasia and/or speech pathologists co-work with mental health professionals to provide services. Whilst this model of delivery will work in some health settings, in others, integrated stroke and mental healthcare pathways do not exist, and there is potential for people with aphasia post stroke to be seen by a number of services in isolation. In practice, only one third of speech pathologists working with people with aphasia report that they frequently train mental health professionals in supportive communication strategies (Sekhon et al., 2015). Further, not all multidisciplinary stroke teams have access to a mental health professional, and specific availability of psychology services is restricted (National Stroke Foundation, 2012). On this account, people with aphasia and mental health problems are at high risk of falling through the cracks. Therefore, there is a strong and urgent need for speech pathologists to engage in this area of clinical need. The principal way this might be achieved is to embed a model within speech pathology practice by which everyone with aphasia accesses the level of support they require. For example, the most recent stroke clinical guidelines in the United Kingdom recommend that psychological care provided by stroke services be based upon three main models of service delivery (collaborative care, matched care and stepped care; Intercollegiate Stroke Working Party, 2016). The model that this article explores further is that of "stepped psychological care" (Kneebone, 2016).

Stepped psychological care

Stepped psychological care after stroke is described as the hierarchical delivery of routine assessment and interventions for emotional difficulties and psychological problems (Kneebone, 2016). This model has been demonstrated to be effective in a range of contexts with varying populations (Firth, Barkham, & Kellett, 2015) and has been applied internationally into various health services (e.g., Australian Department of Health; The National Health Service of Great Britain and Northern Ireland). Stepped psychological care models are based on increasing levels of tailored intervention and have usually been described to either have three or four levels progressing from "low" intensity to "high" intensity interventions (e.g., National Institute for Health and Clinical Excellence, 2009; National Institute for Health and Clinical Excellence, 2011; Kneebone, 2016).

Within the literature, descriptions of stepped psychological care and the level of intervention a person typically first receives vary (Intercollegiate Stroke Working Party, 2016). Kneebone (2016) has provided a narrative review and proposed a model for stepped psychological care after stroke (Figure 1.1). In Kneebone's (2016) stepped psychological care approach, four levels of intervention are described, and a person is matched to the intervention level that most suits their current need. In other words, an individual does not generally have to start at the lowest, least intensive level of intervention to progress to the next "step". Rather, they enter the system and have their service level aligned to their requirements. If at any point their condition deteriorates or if they do not respond to the intervention, they proceed to the next step in the model where the service becomes increasingly tailored and is delivered by more specialised practitioners. Similarly, someone who has benefitted from a higher-level intervention initially might "step down" and maintain their treatment outcome with a less-intensive intervention.

In Kneebone's (2016) stepped psychological care model, level 1 intervention, or the "lowest" intensity intervention, is described as appropriate for all

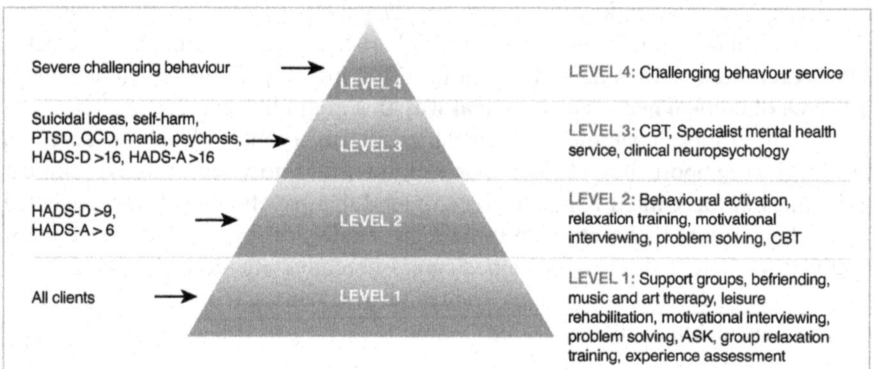

Note: ASK = Action Success Knowledge Program for People with Aphasia, HADS = Hospital Anxiety and Depression Scale, -D Depression subscale, -A Anxiety subscale, CBT = Cognitive Behavioural Therapy, PTSD = Post Traumatic Stress Disorder, OCD = Obsessive Compulsive Disorder.

Figure 1.1 A revised model for stepped psychological care after stroke

Source: Reproduced with permission from Kneebone, 2016

stroke survivors because of the psychological impact of stroke. At this level the therapeutic target is prevention of the onset of mental disorders and treatment of "sub-threshold problems" such as general difficulties with coping and experience of general distress. Level 2 interventions target mild/moderate symptoms of impaired mood. Levels 3 and 4 of the model are for severe and persistent disorders and/or challenging behaviours (Kneebone, 2016).

The role of speech pathologists within stepped psychological care

Potential roles of a speech pathologist within stepped psychological care for people with aphasia may include that of 1) screening for mood problems, 2) provision of low-intensity psychological interventions and 3) facilitation of high-intensity psychological interventions.

Screening for mood problems within stepped psychological care for people with aphasia

A speech pathologist may act as a key worker to carry out screening procedures for people with aphasia and/or provide team-based education on anxiety and depression screening tools specific to people with aphasia. Kneebone's (2016) stepped psychological care model uses the Hospital Anxiety and Depression Scale (HADS; Zigmond & Snaith, 1983) to identify the possible presence and severity of a mood disorder. However, the HADS is a self-report measure and may not always be a suitable assessment tool for people with aphasia because of their communication difficulties. As such, aphasia-specific assessments can be used to assist with identification of mental health problems in this population. To screen for depression in people with aphasia, appropriate tools include the Stroke Aphasic Depression Questionnaire-10 (SADQ-10; Leeds, Meera, & Hobson, 2004), the Stroke Aphasic Depression Questionnaire-Hospital 10 (SADQH-10; Bennett, Thomas, Austen, Morris, & Lincoln, 2006) and the Signs of Depression Scale (SOD; Watkins et al., 2001). These tools have all been recommended for use in clinical practice in a recent systematic review (Van Dijk, De Man-van Ginkel, Hafsteinsdóttir, & Schuurmans, 2016). All three of these tools use observer ratings of behaviour to screen for depression after stroke. The Behavioural Outcomes of Anxiety scale can be used to screen for anxiety in people with aphasia (BOA; Eccles, Morris, & Kneebone, 2017) and, to the best of our knowledge, this is the only instrument that has been validated to screen for symptoms of anxiety in aphasia. The BOA also uses observer ratings of behaviour to identify anxiety after stroke. It is important to remember these instruments in themselves do not diagnose a particular disorder; however, they identify the need for further specialist assessment. Quality of Life assessments specifically designed for use with people with aphasia may also provide information about factors relating to the patient's psychological status. Assessments include the Stroke and Aphasia Quality of Life Scale (SAQoL-39; Hilari, Byng, Lamping, & Smith, 2003) and the Assessment for Living with Aphasia (ALA; Kagan et al., 2011). Both of these assessments are self-report measures.

It important to note that while screening is recommended in guidance (e.g., Stroke Foundation Australian Clinical Guidelines for Stroke Management, 2017), it is unknown if such an assessment improves outcomes (Towfighi et al., 2017). But it seems sensible that routine screening should form part of a broader formal clinical pathway which includes follow-up mood assessment and intervention procedures for people with aphasia (Lincoln et al., 2012).

Provision of lower intensity psychological interventions

Communicatively accessible psychoeducation could be developed by a speech pathologist in consultation with the multidisciplinary team and routinely provided as part of stroke care. Psychoeducation topics could include ways to cope and manage with the impact of aphasia, signs and symptoms of mental health problems, and contacts for further services and/or support if required. In addition to psychoeducation, access to counselling services may be helpful regardless of the presence or absence of mood disorder. Speech pathologists may develop co-work models of intervention so that generic counselling delivered by stroke professionals is communicatively accessible for people with aphasia as well as training mental health practitioners in supported conversation techniques. It is important to note that speech pathologists report using a range of counselling techniques for people with aphasia post stroke but are not always confident to do so (see Sekhon et al., 2015); hence additional training may be required.

A speech pathologist may integrate stepped psychological care intervention into speech pathology sessions for people with aphasia and their families. The purpose of this intervention would be to prevent deterioration of emotional wellbeing and provide strategies to enhance mood (within the scope of their skills and qualifications). According to practice guidelines in Australia, it is within the scope of a speech pathologist's role to provide mental health treatment but it considered an advanced area of practice that requires specialist knowledge. If the level of intervention needed is not within scope of practice, a speech pathologist may also coordinate referral to an experienced mental health practitioner trained to work with people with aphasia or develop models of co-work. Baker et al. (2018) have conducted a systematic review of the evidence-based interventions for people with aphasia within the stepped psychological care model after stroke. The review considered the research evidence available for psychological and other stroke rehabilitation interventions specifically for people with aphasia. In the Baker et al. (2018) review, interventions were classified as either 1) preventive interventions that target those at high risk of depression after stroke or 2) treatment interventions that target those who fulfil criteria for depression after stroke or 3) stroke rehabilitation interventions that indirectly targeted depression as an outcome through stroke rehabilitation. From this review it was identified that level 1 intervention within stepped psychological care for people with aphasia with sub-threshold symptoms may include:

- Goal setting related to participation goals specific to targeting depression through a multimodal stroke intervention, including telephone contacts, screening for adverse sequelae, written information, home visits, review of goal achievement and further referral to relevant health services
  (Graven, Brock, Hill, Cotton, & Joubert, 2016)
- Completion of self-management workbook(s) based on self-efficacy principles used for a period of four weeks
  (Jones, Mandy, & Partridge, 2009)
- Biographic-narrative therapy focussed on identity redevelopment through one-on-one narrative interviews and group intervention
  (Corsten, Schimpf, Konradi, Keilmann, & Hardering, 2015)
- Psychosocial group support focused on sharing of personal experience with other people with aphasia
  (Brumfitt & Sheeran, 1997)
- Participation in a community choir comprising other people with aphasia
  (Tamplin, Baker, Jones, Way, & Lee, 2013)

Additional level 1 treatment options that may also be considered for people with aphasia that have been found to have some evidence for their use include:

- Aphasia Action Success and Knowledge (ASK) therapy – a packaged program that incorporates goal setting, psychoeducation and support to help manage the impacts of aphasia
  (Ryan et al., 2017)
- Solution-focussed brief therapy – an approach to building change through encouraging a person to describe their preferred future; exploring a person's skills, resources, resilience and past successes, and enabling people to notice positive signs of change
  (Northcott, Burns, Simpson, & Hilari, 2015)
- Modified motivational interviewing – a talk-based therapy used to help a person understand the importance of changing what they make of their situation
  (Holland, Watkins, Boaden & Lightbody, 2017)

It should be noted that both modified motivational interviewing and solution-focussed brief therapy may also be suitable level 2 stepped psychological care treatments for people with aphasia classified with mild/moderate symptoms of impaired mood; however, to the authors' knowledge, sufficient research evidence for this level of care is not available to date.

Level 2 interventions identified by Baker et al. (2018) within stepped psychological care for people with aphasia with mild to moderate symptoms of mood disorder may include:

- Modified behavioural activation – a treatment focussed on maximizing mood-elevating activities through education, activity monitoring, activity scheduling and graded task assignments

(Thomas, Walker, Macniven, Haworth, & Lincoln, 2013)

Another level 2 treatment option that may also be considered for people with aphasia that has been found to have some evidence for its use includes relaxation training using a self-help relaxation CD (Golding, Kneebone, & Fife-Schaw, 2016; Golding, Fife-Schaw, & Kneebone, 2017, 2018).

Facilitation of higher-intensity psychological interventions

At levels 3 and 4 of stepped psychological care, a speech pathologist may co-work with mental health practitioners to inform mental health diagnosis using clinical interview and assess suicide risk (Townend et al., 2007). Communication support tools could be developed to be used alongside instruments such as the Australian Psychological Society Suicide Risk Assessment Tool (Hawgood & de Leo, 2015; Hawgood & de Leo, 2016) to determine suicide risk (see Butow et al., 2015). If a medication plan is relevant, it may also be important to ensure that it is in a communication-accessible format. To the best of our knowledge, no high-level evidence is available for psychological treatments for people with aphasia at levels 3 and 4 of the stepped care model (Baker et al., 2018). Kneebone and Jeffries (2013) have successfully used modified cognitive-behavioural psychotherapy for anxiety with a person with aphasia, but evidence is only at the case study level.

To illustrate how speech pathologists might work within the stepped care model, a case example, Ben (not his real name), is presented next.

Case study: Ben

Ben is a 55-year-old male. Ben worked full time as a manager in a demanding office-based job where most weeks he worked more than 50 hours. Ben had been married to his wife, Eleanor, for 25 years. They had no children. Eleanor worked part time as a sales assistant in retail. Ben always made an effort to see a close group of friends every week and had a passion for cars and travel. Ben's medical history included hypertension but otherwise Ben was fit, active, social and considered overall healthy. Ben and Eleanor led busy lives and often enjoyed activities independent of each other. Ben sustained a left middle cerebral artery infarct which resulted in moderate to severe fluent aphasia. He had mild physical issues though he was independent with all personal and domestic activities. With respect to communication, Ben found it very difficult to understand others and organise his words in order to be understood. Despite being able to easily say many words, these were often nonsense words. Ben had preserved intonation of voice, body language and facial expressions; however, his language impairment amounted to a severe communication disability. Because of his aphasia, Ben found it particularly difficult to concentrate during conversation and was exhausted after most interactions with others. He suffered ongoing headaches which were also a major source of distress for him. Ben spent 10 days in bed-based hospital care (acute and inpatient rehabilitation service) and was then discharged home. He then received four weeks of interdisciplinary intensive rehabilitation via an early supported discharge program, followed by eight weeks of one to two weekly sessions of community rehabilitation. As Ben reached his maximum length of community rehabilitation, he was discharged on to relevant community services with follow-up appointments to outpatient specialist stroke and speech pathology services. Table 1.1 describes adverse sequelae and psychological issues faced by Ben and Eleanor within each of the rehabilitation services and actions his treating speech pathologist took in the context of Kneebone's (2016) stepped psychological care model.

Table 1.1 Case study of Ben, a person with aphasia after stroke, and services provided by his speech pathologist within a stepped psychological care model. *SADQ-H10* = Stroke Aphasic Depression Questionnaire – Hospital 10 item.

Stroke recovery timeline	*Sources of distress and depression screening results*	*Actions taken by speech pathologist working within stepped psychological care model*
Bed-based hospital care	Ben is agitated and distressed when challenged by "the fast pace" of the hospital Ben appears to be in disbelief about what has happened and repeatedly questions "Why?" SADQ-H10 screening indicates that a possible mood disorder may be present	Respond to specific patient concerns, provide communicatively accessible psychoeducation about stroke and aphasia (level 1 stepped psychological care) Raise concern of Ben's distress and possible mood decline in SP clinical notes in patient file, at ward case conference meeting and to charge nurse. Flag review with medical team +/− referral to psychologist. Document the outcome of the SADQ-H10 screening on handover to the early discharge stroke service

(Continued)

Table 1.1 (Continued)

Stroke recovery timeline	*Sources of distress and depression screening results*	*Actions taken by speech pathologist working within stepped psychological care model*
Intensive interdisciplinary in-home rehabilitation	Re-screening using the SADQH-10 tool indicates that a possible mood disorder may be present Ben's wife reports she is concerned about the changes in Ben's behavior. She reports he does not want to do his speech therapy tasks, gets angry with her quickly and she does not know how to help him. Ben's words become worse when he is distressed which seems to be often, and he often expresses the word 'useless'. Where previously he enjoyed his fiends visiting, Ben is declining all visitors. Ben is declining friend visits	Discussion of SADQ-H10 screening results with Ben and his wife Provision of information about options of support at low-intensity psychological stepped care levels Co-work with social worker with the aim to normalise the need to seek help after stroke Referral for Ben to a stroke group (level 1 stepped psychological care)
Community rehabilitation	Ben's wife reports a further decline in his mood, and interest in 'doing anything'. Ben's affect is noticeably flat and he is difficult to motivate in speech therapy. His communication attempts are less and he continues to express the word 'useless' in therapy. Re-screening using the SADQ-H10 indicates a decline in mood that would warrant consideration of higher levels of stepped psychological care	Discussion of SADQ-H10 screening results with Ben and his wife Co-work with the community psychologist to provide behavioural activation treatment. The aim of behavioural activation is to increase the level of meaningful and enjoyable activity in order to improve mood (Thomas et al., 2013; level 2 of stepped psychological care) As Ben's mood improved/declined, on-going mood management within stepped psychological care would be "stepped up" or "stepped down" as required

Discussion

In this chapter we have presented a case study, Ben that demonstrates an opportunity for speech pathologists to take up a leadership role and support people with aphasia to access mental health treatments. Stepped psychological care after stroke is a relatively new model of mental health service provision that has the potential to improve access to psychological care for people with aphasia. The success of the model, however, is dependent on a number of factors. First and foremost, the suggestions included in this article would need to be further developed and validated into a formal clinical pathway for the psychological management of people with post-stroke aphasia. This is particularly important given that clinical guidelines and pathways are used as a main source of research evidence by speech pathologists to inform aphasia management (Verna, Davidson, & Rose, 2009). Such a clinical pathway may provide guidance on specific timelines for both assessment and interventions within the stepped psychological care model as well as clarifying the roles of other multidisciplinary team stroke members. For example, detailed clinical pathways that clarify timing, professional roles and content of interventions within a stepped psychological care model already exist for cancer care (Butow et al., 2015). If a psychological care model is to be introduced into "usual care", the role of both speech pathologists and other multidisciplinary team stroke members may also be considered in light of the NHS Improvement Stroke recommendations (Gillham & Clarke, 2011). These recommendations offer a practice guide for how a service might implement stepped psychological care.

Successful implementation of a stepped psychological care model would also require consideration of associated costs and workforce implications. Future research investigating the efficacy and cost effectiveness of the model compared with "usual care" is warranted. This would include the costs of speech pathologists receiving the necessary training to incorporate appropriate stepped psychological care interventions into their everyday practice. It is important that speech pathologists feel not only competent but also confident to work within the mental health arena at a level appropriate to their training and professional boundaries. Hence, professional development opportunities would also need to be provided. Workforce implications such as the impact on the capacity for staff to continue fulfilling more traditional speech pathologist roles would also need to be considered. It may be that the introduction of such a model may not drastically change how much time speech pathologists are spending to improve the psychological wellbeing of people with aphasia but may improve how effective they are in doing so.

Conclusion

The delivery of psychological care to people with aphasia and their families is unique because of the impact of communication difficulties and the skills required by health care personnel to provide support, optimise health care interactions and access to treatment. Speech pathologists are well positioned to contribute to the psychological care for people with aphasia, often taking on the role of communication broker between a person with aphasia and the stroke team. However, there is a paucity of service models to support them in this endeavour. Stepped psychological care provides a framework for all stroke healthcare professionals to take responsibility and provide psychological care as able. In this article we have outlined the particular role a speech pathologist may take within the model.

This article is a call for speech pathologists to step up to the existing and growing needs of this vulnerable population of people with aphasia. In this paper, we have offered one possible solution of a new model of care. We recognise that, to implement stepped psychological care for people with aphasia, speech pathologists will require systemic support, relevant training for effective practice, and clear practice guidelines and pathways. The evidence of the incidence of depression and anxiety for people with aphasia is irrefutable. Therefore, we hope to move the conversation from the debate about whether or not speech pathologists should work in this space to how the profession can move forward in enabling psychological wellbeing, ultimately improving the lives of people with aphasia and their families.

Notes

1 "Speech pathologist" is the term used in Australia. It is acknowledged that in some other countries, including the UK, the term used is "speech and language therapist".
2 School of Health and Rehabilitation Sciences, The University of Queensland, Australia
3 School of Allied Health, College of Science, Health and Engineering, La Trobe University, Australia
4 Faculty of Health Sciences, The University of Sydney, Australia
5 Health and Human Sciences, Southeastern Louisiana University, United States
6 Discipline of Clinical Psychology, Graduate School of Health, University of Technology, Sydney, Australia
7 Centre of Research Excellence in Aphasia Recovery and Rehabilitation, Australia

References

Baker, C., Worrall, L., Rose, M., Ryan, B., Hudson, K., & O'Byrne, L. (2018). A systematic review of rehabilitation interventions to prevent and treat depression in post-stroke aphasia. *Disability and Rehabilitation*, *40*(16), 1870–1892. https://doi.org/10.1080/09638288.2017.1315181

Bennett, H. E., Thomas, S. A., Austen, R., Morris, A. M. S., & Lincoln, N. B. (2006). Validation of screening measures for assessing mood in stroke patients. *British Journal of Clinical Psychology*, *45*(3), 367–376. https://doi.org/10.1348/014466505X58277

Brady, M. C., Fredrick, A., & Williams, B. (2013). People with aphasia: Capacity to consent, research participation and intervention inequalities. *International Journal of Stroke*, *8*(3), 193–196. https://doi.org/10.1111/j.1747-4949.2012.00900.x

Brown, K., Worrall, L., Davidson, B., & Howe, T. (2010). Snapshots of success: An insider perspective on living successfully with aphasia. *Aphasiology*, *24*, 1267–1295.

Brumfitt, S. (1993). Losing your sense of self: What aphasia can do. *Aphasiology*, *7*(6), 569–575.

Brumfitt, S. (2006). Psychosocial aspects of aphasia: Speech and language therapists' view on professional practice. *Disability and Rehabilitation*, *28*(8), 523–534.

Brumfitt, S., & Sheeran, P. (1997). An evaluation of short-term group therapy for people with aphasia. *Disability and Rehabilitation*, *19*(6), 221–230.

Butow, P., Price, M. A., Shaw, J. M., Turner, J., Clayton, J. M., Grimison, P. . . . Kirsten, L. (2015). Clinical pathway for the screening, assessment and management of anxiety and depression in adult cancer patients: Australian guidelines. *Psycho-Oncology*, *24*(9), 987–1001. https://doi.org/10.1002/pon.3920

Campbell, G. B., Skidmore, E. R., Whyte, E. M., & Matthews, J. T. (2015). Overcoming practical challenges to conducting clinical research in the inpatient stroke rehabilitation setting. *Topics in Stroke Rehabilitation*, *22*(5), 386–394. https://doi.org/10.1179/1074935714Z.0000000045

Carota, A., Staub, F., & Bogousslavsky, J. (2002). Emotions, behaviours and mood changes in stroke. *Current Opinion in Neurology*, *15*, 57–69.

Code, C., & Herrmann, M. (2003). The relevance of emotional and psychosocial factors in aphasia to rehabilitation. *Neuropsychological Rehabilitation*, *13*(1–2), 109–132.

Corsten, S., Schimpf, E. J., Konradi, J., Keilmann, A., & Hardering, F. (2015). The participants' perspective: How biographic-narrative intervention influences identity negotiation and quality of life in aphasia. *International Journal of Language & Communication Disorders*, *50*(6), 788.

Cruice, M., Hill, R., Worrall, L., & Hickson, L. (2010). Conceptualising quality of life for older people with aphasia. *Aphasiology*, *24*, 327–345.

Cruice, M., Worrall, L., & Hickson, L. (2011). Reporting on psychological well-being of older adults with chronic aphasia in the context of unaffected peers. *Disability and Rehabilitation: An International, Multidisciplinary Journal*, *33*(3), 219–228.

Cruice, M., Worrall, L., Hickson, L., & Murison, R. (2003). Finding a focus for quality of life with aphasia: Social and emotional health, and psychological well-being. *Aphasiology*, *17*, 333–353.

Dalemans, R., Wade, D. T., van den Heuvel, W. J. A., & de Witte, L. P. (2009). Facilitating the participation of people with aphasia in research: A description of strategies. *Clinical Rehabilitation*, *23*, 948–959.

Deloitte Access Economics. (2013). *The economic impact of stroke in Australia*. Sydney, Australia: Deloitte Access Economics.

Eccles, A., Morris, R., & Kneebone, I. (2017). Psychometric properties of the Behavioural Outcomes of Anxiety Questionnaire in stroke patients with aphasia. *Clinical Rehabilitation*, *31*(3), 369–378.

Firth, N., Barkham, M., & Kellett, S. (2015). The clinical effectiveness of stepped care systems for depression in working age adults: A systematic review. *Journal of Affective Disorders*, *170*, 119–130.

Flowers, H. L., Skoretz, S. A., Silver, F. L., Rochon, E., Fang, J., Flamand-Roze, C., & Martino, R. (2016). Poststroke aphasia frequency, recovery and outcomes: A systematic review and meta-analysis. *Archives of Physical Medicine and Rehabilitation*, *97*, 2188–2201. https://doi.org/10.1016/j.apmr.2016.03.006

Fucetola, R., Connor, L. T., Perry, J., Leo, P., Tucker, F. M., & Corbetta, M. (2006). Aphasia severity, semantics, and depression predict functional communication in acquired aphasia. *Aphasiology*, *20*(5), 449–461.

Gillham, S., & Clarke, L. (2011). *Psychological care after stroke: Improving stroke services for people with cognitive and mood disorders*. Leicester: NHS Improvement.

Golding, K., Fife-Schaw, C., & Kneebone, I. I. (2018). A pilot randomised controlled trial of self-help relaxation to reduce post-stroke depression. *Clinical Rehabilitation*, *32*, 747–751. doi:10.1177/02692155177419

Golding, K., Fife-Schaw, C., & Kneebone, I. I. (2017). Twelve month follow-up on a randomised controlled trial of relaxation training for post-stroke anxiety. *Clinical Rehabilitation*, *31*, 1164–1167 doi:10.1177/0269215516682820

Golding, K., Kneebone, I., & Fife-Schaw, C. (2016). Self-help relaxation for post-stroke anxiety: A randomised, controlled pilot study. *Clinical Rehabilitation, 30*, 174–180. doi:10.1177/0269215515575746

Graven, C. D., Brock, K., Hill, K., Cotton, S., & Joubert, L. (2016). First year after stroke: An integrated approach focusing on participation goals aiming to reduce depressive symptoms. *Stroke, 47*(11), 2820–2827.

Hackett, M., Anderson, C., House, A., & Halteh, C. (2008). Interventions for preventing depression after stroke. *Cochrane Database Systematic Reviews, 3*. https://doi.org/10.1002/14651858.CD003689.Pub3.

Hallowell, B., & Chapey, R. (2008). Introduction to language intervention strategies in adult aphasia. In R. Chapey (Ed.), *Language intervention strategies in aphasia and related neurogenic communication disorders* (5th ed., pp. 3–19). Philadelphia, PA: Lippincott Williams & Wilkins.

Hawgood, J., & de Leo, D. (2015). *STARS: Screening tool for assessing risk of suicide*. Brisbane: Australian Institute for Suicide Research and Prevention, Griffith University.

Hawgood, J., & de Leo, D. (2016). Reconceptualising suicide risk assessment: A person-centred approach to needs-based exploration of current suicidality. *InPsych: The Bulletin of the Australian Psychological Society Ltd, 38*, 10.

Hilari, K., & Byng, S. (2009). Health-related quality of life in people with severe aphasia. *International Journal of Language & Communication Disorders, 44*(2), 193–205. https://doi.org/10.1080/13682820802008820

Hilari, K., Byng, S., Lamping, D., & Smith, S. (2003). Stroke and aphasia quality of life scale-39 (SAQOL-39). *Stroke, 34*, 1944–1950.

Hilari, K., Needle, J. J., & Harrison, K. L. (2012). What are the important factors in health-related quality of life for people with aphasia? A systematic review. *Archives of Physical Medicine & Rehabilitation, 93*(1), S86–S95. https://doi.org/10.1016/j.apmr.2011.05.028

Hilari, K., Wiggins, R., Roy, P., Byng, S., & Smith, S. (2003). Predictors of Health-related Quality of Life (HRQL) in people with chronic aphasia. *Aphasiology, 17*(4), 365–381. https://doi.org/10.1080/02687030244000725

Holland, E., Watkins, C., Boaden, E., & Lightbody, C. (2017). Fidelity to a motivational interviewing intervention for those with post-stroke aphasia: A small-scale feasibility study. *Topics in Stroke Rehabilitation*, 1–7.

Intercollegiate Stroke Working Party. (2016). *National clinical guidelines for stroke* (5th ed.) [Online]. London. Retrieved 28 November 2017 from www.strokeaudit.org/SupportFiles/Documents/Guidelines/2016-National-Clinical-Guideline-for-Stroke-5t-(1).aspx

Jones, F., Mandy, A., & Partridge, C. (2009). Changing self-efficacy in individuals following a first time stroke: Preliminary study of a novel self-management intervention. *Clinical Rehabilitation, 23*(6), 522–533.

Kagan, A., Simmons-Mackie, N., Victor, J. C., Carling-Rowland, A., Hoch, J., Huijbregts, M. . . . Mok, A. (2011). *Assessment for Living with Aphasia (ALA)*. Toronto, ON: Aphasia Institute.

Kauhanen, M., Korperlainen, J. T., Hiltunen, P., Maatta, R., Mononen, H., Brusin, E. . . . Myllyla, V. V. (2000). Aphasia, depression, and non-verbal cognitive impairment in ischaemic stroke. *Cerebrovascular Disease, 10*, 455–461.

Kneebone, I. I. (2016). Stepped psychological care after stroke. *Disability and Rehabilitation, 38*(18), 1836.

Kneebone, I. I., & Jeffries, F. W. (2013). Treating anxiety after stroke using cognitive behaviour therapy: Two cases. *Neuropsychological Rehabilitation, 23*, 798–810. https://doi.org/10.1080/09602011.2013.820135

Kutlubaev, M. A., & Hackett, M. L. (2014). Part II: Predictors of depression after stroke and impact of depression on stroke outcome: An updated systematic review of observational studies. *International Journal of Stroke, 9*, 1026–1036.

LaFond, D. (Ed.). (1993). *Living with aphasia: Psychosocial issues*. San Diego, CA: Singular Publishing Group.

Leeds, L., Meera, R. J., & Hobson, J. F. (2004). The utility of the Stroke Aphasia Depression Questionnaire in a stroke rehabilitation unit. *Clinical Rehabilitation, 18*, 228–231.

Lincoln, N., & Kneebone, I. I. (2012). Psychological problems after stroke and their management: State of knowledge. *Neuroscience & Medicine, 3*, 83–89.

Lincoln, N., Kneebone, I. I., Macniven, J., & Morris, R. (2012). *Psychological management of stroke*. Chichester: Wiley.

Menlove, L., Crayton, E., Kneebone, I., Allen-Crooks, R., Otto, E., & Harder, H. (2015). Predictors of anxiety after stroke: A systematic review of observational studies. *Journal of Stroke and Cerebrovascular Diseases, 24*, 1107–1117.

Morris, R., Eccles, A., Ryan, B., & Kneebone, I. (2017). Prevalence of anxiety in people with aphasia after stroke. *Aphasiology, 31*(12), 1410–1415. https://doi.org/10.1080/02687038.2017.1304633

National Institute for Health and Clinical Excellence. (2009). *Depression: Management of depression in primary and secondary healthcare*. London: National Institute for Health and Clinical Excellence.

National Institute for Health and Clinical Excellence. (2011). *Generalised anxiety disorder and panic (with or without agoraphobia) in adults*. London: National Institute for Health and Clinical Excellence.

National Stroke Foundation. (2012). *National stroke audit: Rehabilitation services report*. Melbourne: National Stroke Foundation.

Northcott, S., Burns, K., Simpson, A., & Hilari, K. (2015). 'Living with aphasia the best way I can': A feasibility study exploring solution-focused brief therapy for people with aphasia. *Folia Phoniatrica Et Logopaedica, 67*(3), 156–167.

Northcott, S., Simpson, A., Moss, B., Ahmed, N., & Hilari, K. (2016). How do speech-and-language therapists address the psychosocial well-being of people with aphasia? Results of a UK online survey: Addressing psychosocial needs following aphasia. *International Journal of Language & Communication, 52*(3), 356–373.

Parr, S. (2001). Psychosocial aspects of aphasia: Whose perspectives? *Folia Phoniatrica et Logopaedica, 53*(5), 266–288.

Ryan, B., Hudson, K., Worrall, L., Simmons-Mackie, N., Thomas, E., Finch, K., . . . Lethlean, B. (2017). The aphasia action, success, and knowledge programme: Results from an Australian phase I trial of a speech-pathology-led intervention for people with aphasia early post stroke. *Brain Impairment, 18*(3), 284–298. https://doi.org/10.1017/BrImp.2017.5

Ryan, B., Bohan, J., & Kneebone, I. (2019). Help-seeking and people with aphasia who have mood problems after stroke: Perspectives of speech–language pathologists. *International Journal of Language & Communication Disorders, 54*(5), 779–793. https://doi.org/10.1111/1460-6984.12476

Robinson, R. (2010). Neuropsychiatric disorders following stroke. *Canadian Journal of Psychiatry, 55*(6), 339–340.

Sekhon, J., Douglas, J., & Rose, M. (2015). Current Australian speech-language pathology practice in addressing psychological well-being in people with aphasia after stroke. *International Journal of Speech-Language Pathology, 17*(3), 252–262.

Shadden, B., Hagstrom, F., & Koski, P. (2008). *Neurogenic communication disorders: Life stories and the narrative self.* San Diego, CA: Plural Publishing.

Stroke Foundation. (2018). *National stroke audit: Rehabilitation services report.* Melbourne: Stroke Foundation. Retrieved from https://informme.org.au/stroke-data/Rehabilitation-audits

Tamplin, J., Baker, F. A., Jones, B., Way, A., & Lee, S. (2013). 'Stroke a chord': The effect of singing in a community choir on mood and social engagement for people living with aphasia following a stroke. *NeuroRehabilitation, 32*(4), 929–941.

Tanner, D. (2003). Eclectic perspectives on the psychology of aphasia. *Journal of Allied Health, 32*(4), 256.

Thomas, S. A., & Lincoln, N. B. (2006). Factors relating to depression after stroke. *British Journal of Clinical Psychology, 45*(1), 49–61.

Thomas, S. A., Walker, M. F., Macniven, J. A., Haworth, H., & Lincoln, N. B. (2013). Communication and Low Mood (CALM): A randomized controlled trial of behavioural therapy for stroke patients with aphasia. *Clinical Rehabilitation, 27*, 398–408.

Towfighi, A. L., Ovbiagele, B. E., El Husseini, N. M., Hackett, M. H., Jorge, R. A., Kissela, B. S. . . . Williams, L. (2017). Poststroke depression: A scientific statement for healthcare professionals from the American Heart Association/American Stroke Association. *Stroke, 48*(2), E30–E43.

Townend, E., Brady, M., & McLaughlan, K. (2007). Exclusion and inclusion criteria for people with aphasia in studies of depression after stroke: A systematic review and future recommendations. *Neuroepidemiology*, 29, 1–17.

Van Dijk, M., De Man-van Ginkel, J., Hafsteinsdóttir, T., & Schuurmans, M. (2016). Identifying depression post-stroke in patients with aphasia: A systematic review of the reliability, validity and feasibility of available instruments. *Clinical Rehabilitation, 30*(8), 795–810.

Verna, A., Davidson, B., & Rose, T. (2009). Speech-language pathology services for people with aphasia: A survey of current practice in Australia. *International Journal of Speech-Language Pathology, 11*(3), 191–205.

Watkins, C., Leathley, M., Daniels, L., Dickinson, H., Lightbody, C. E., van den Broek, M., & Jack, C. I. A. (2001). The signs of depression scale in stroke. *Clinical Rehabilitation, 15*, 456.

Worrall, L. E., Hudson, K., Khan, A., Ryan, B., & Simmons-Mackie, N. (2017). Determinants of living well with aphasia in the first year poststroke: A prospective cohort study. *Archives of Physical Medicine and Rehabilitation, 98*(2), 235–240.

Zigmond, A. S., & Snaith, R. P. (1983). The hospital anxiety and depression scale. *Acta Psychiatrica Scandinavica, 67*, 361–370.

Chapter 2

The importance of syntax in making meaning and emotional adjustment

A brief psychodynamically oriented intervention in receptive aphasia

Aonghus Ryan

> The word is a complex neuropsychological entity – comprised of numerous component parts – each of which plays a different role in the functional organisation of the mental apparatus.
>
> (Kaplan-Solms and Solms, 2000, pp. 90–91)

Patients with neurological damage can face many challenges in adjusting to the sudden personal and social losses which frequently accompany neurological injury, and certain cognitive problems can further complicate the process of adjustment. Limited insight into deficits, changes in how emotions are experienced and concrete thinking can alter the process of normal grieving – sometimes referred to as *normal mourning* (Salas & Coetzer, 2015). Particular problems with language can also adversely affect emotional adjustment, as this chapter attempts to illustrate. Language is understood in psychoanalytic metapsychology as enabling humans to bring the unconscious mental processes of the ego into conscious awareness through auditory-verbal associations and abstractions, by attaching words to thoughts. Freud posited that it is specifically the auditory-verbal element of words, not their motor or visual representations, that is crucial in reliably bringing the ego's processes into conscious awareness: "In essence a word is after all the mnemic residue of a word *heard*" (Freud, 1923b). Freud's emphasis on the word "heard" raises questions about the effect deficits in receptive language may have on patients' conscious awareness.

Of course, language involves more than understanding individual word meanings; it goes beyond semantics. Syntax (e.g., grammar, prepositions and conjunctives) is the discrete combinatorial system of language enabling us to make practically infinite connections (Pinker, 1994). Semantics and syntax are not independent of each other; indeed, Caplan, Hildebrandt, and Marshall (1988) highlighted the importance of achieving access to the syntactico-semantic representations of words for comprehension in receptive aphasia. Solms also indirectly drew our attention to the importance of syntax: "what is most important about words is their capacity to represent the relations between things, to re-represent them abstractly. This enables us to think *about* things as opposed to merely think things. . . . In short, words enable us to think about the relations between things both in space and in time" (Solms, 2013, pp. 14–15). The possibilities conferred by the syntax of language to hold steady in mind an array of interconnected ideas allows the emergence of new ideas, connections and solutions. In other words, syntax supports the mental process of sifting through ideas to find deeper meaning. Indeed, bringing unconscious mental processes into conscious awareness to reflect on our thoughts by attaching words to thoughts – *reflexive consciousness* – through the semantics and syntax of language is one of the key mechanisms of change in psychotherapy, hence the "talking cure" (Solms, 2013).

It follows that changes in our ability to attach words to thoughts through language, and therefore to reflect about things in time and in space, have implications for emotional adjustment in neurological rehabilitation. More specifically, deficits in syntactic understanding might reduce patients' capacity to engage in the deep meaning-making crucial to normal mourning. In considering such deeper sense-making, we are pushing the limits of language to describe the human condition, entering the realm of the arts, literature and poetry. Perhaps unsurprisingly, writing has long been viewed as a useful compensatory strategy in neurological rehabilitation, particularly to compensate for deficits in attention and memory (Luria, 1963). There is also some evidence that poetry can be useful in processing emotions in neurological rehabilitation (Prigatano, Borgaro, & Caples, 2003).

Two of Luria's seven types of aphasia – acoustico-mnestic aphasia and semantic aphasia – are relevant for the current case, Ms A, and a relevant case study, Mrs K (Kaplan-Solms & Solms, 2000, see later). First, Luria's acoustico-mnestic aphasia (also known as *amnestic aphasia*) is defined as difficulty in retaining word series or grasping full sentences, not a deficit in understanding individual word meanings (Whitworth, Webster, & Howard, 2005). Another way to conceptualise acoustico-mnestic aphasia is as a deficit in auditory-verbal working memory – an inability to stabilise auditory-verbal traces (Francis, Clark, & Humphreys, 2003; Kaplan-Solms & Solms, 2000). Second, Luria's semantic aphasia is defined as a "disturbance in the understanding of logico-grammatical relationships . . . characterised by an inability to synthesise isolated simultaneous events into a meaningful unity" (Whitworth et al., 2005, p. 69). As with acoustico-mnestic aphasia, the meaning of single words is intact in semantic aphasia; however, there are often object-naming and spatial orientation difficulties. So, in some ways, the name "semantic aphasia" is confusing, as it encompasses both semantics and syntax.

The specific effects of acoustico-mnestic aphasia on emotional adjustment in neurological rehabilitation were explored by Kaplan-Solms and Solms (2000), who reported the case of Mrs K, who was "unable to attach words to her thoughts, and therefore, unable to render her thoughts conscious" (Kaplan-Solms & Solms, 2000, p. 108). This was subjectively experienced by Mrs K as an "inability to think". Kaplan-Solms and Solms coined the term *perforated consciousness*: fundamental problems in reflexive consciousness caused by reduced abilities to make auditory-verbal associations or to generate repeating synaptic firing patterns to stabilise information in the mind. Consequences for Mrs K included difficulties in making sense of the world, undermined self-identity, and a delay in engaging in normal mourning for the many losses she had experienced (Kaplan-Solms & Solms, 2000). However, the case of Mrs K did not shed light on how changes in the ability to think about the relations between things – through syntax – affect deeper meaning-making, self-awareness and emotional adjustment after brain injury.

Speech and language therapy

In the UK, speech and language therapists (SLTs) work most closely with patients with aphasia. Two assessments which consider syntax by assessing sentence comprehension and receptive grammar are the *Psycholinguistic Assessments of Language Assessments in Aphasia* (PALPA; Kay, Lesser, & Coltheart, 1992), and Bishop's (1989) *Test for the Reception of Grammar* (TROG). Anecdotally, both the PALPA and the TROG are less frequently used than the Pyramids and Palm Trees Test (Howard & Patterson, 1992), based on the widely used Patterson and Shewell's (1987) model (Figure 2.1.). This model separates the phonological (spoken and heard) and orthographical (seen and written) aspects of single words, with a centrally placed semantic system containing all the related concepts to word meaning. A notable limitation of this commonly used model is its focus on single words and the absence of syntax and grammatical structures understood to be a factor in the verbal communicative ability of aphasic patients (Doesborgh, 2004).

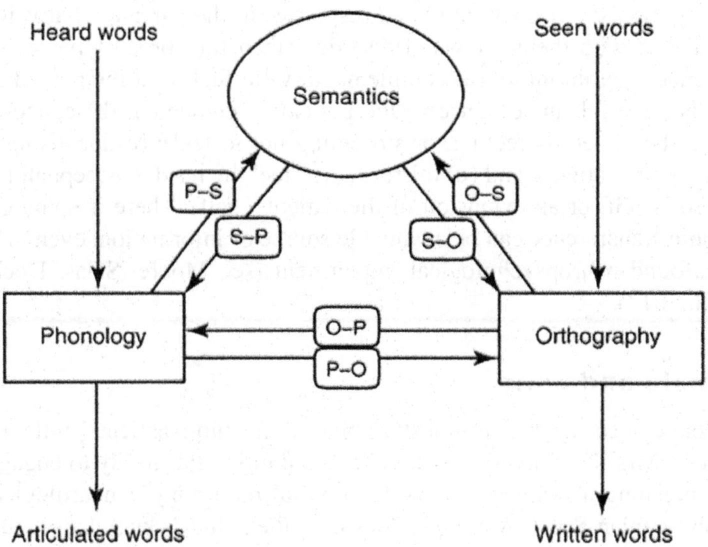

Figure 2.1 A cognitive model of single-word processing
Source: Patterson & Shewell, 1987

There are a number of treatment approaches for receptive aphasia, including: *comprehension training*, which aims to help the patient focus more on listening and comprehension rather than focusing on speech production; *stimulation training*, aiming to promote other areas of the brain, particularly the frontal lobes, to compensate for comprehension through sustained exposure to verbal stimulation; and the *social approach*, which focuses principally on maximising functional communication (LaPointe, 2005). Four syntax-based aphasia therapy studies were reviewed systematically by Horan (2016), suggesting mixed outcomes for each of the studies included. More recently, researchers have begun to conceptualise receptive aphasia as a deficit in auditory-verbal working memory; however, several small studies aimed at improving sentence comprehension using this theoretical approach have also yielded mixed results (Salis, Hwang, Howard, & Lallini, 2017).

Clinical neuropsychology

Language deficits present several challenges in gathering the kinds of data which clinical neuropsychologists draw on to formulate a patient's presentation, particularly as most standard neuropsychological assessments rely on receptive language ability to understand test instructions. Direct clinical interview is generally less precise, and the clinician will often employ aphasia-friendly neuropsychological assessments and psychometrics, observation in functional settings, behavioural analysis and information from family members. A less frequently considered yet potentially valuable source of data is countertransference in working with neurological patients: our own emotional responses to the patient, what it feels like to spend time with them. Lewis (1999) described four broad types of countertransference in brain injury (a) complementary (to feel what the patient's family or friends have felt in response to the patient's behaviour); (b) concordant (to feel what the patient is feeling, or struggling not to feel); (c) idealising (to feel admired by the patient); and (d) mirroring (to feel the need to accept and confirm the patient's self, or an extension of the patient's self). There is some evidence that countertransference can be a valuable source of information, even in patients with profound neuropsychological impairment (see Moore, Salas, Dockree, & Turnbull, 2017).

Rationale and aims

As we have seen, acoustico-mnestic aphasia can limit patients' reflexive consciousness, Mrs K's "inability to think", thus limiting the ability to engage in the kind of meaning-making necessary for normal mourning in neurological rehabilitation (Kaplan-Solms & Solms, 2000). To the author's knowledge, such deficits in reflexive consciousness and their potential effects on normal mourning are likely to be unfamiliar to most SLTs and clinical neuropsychologists in the UK. Given that understanding the logico-grammatical rules of language (syntax) are a core feature of Luria's semantic aphasia and given that syntax is understood to allow for cortical programming, planning and sequencing (Solms, 2013), it is possible that the role of receptive language ability and syntax in meaning-making and emotional adjustment in neurological rehabilitation has been overlooked, and that the deficits in reflexive consciousness seen in acoustic-mnestic aphasia may be understood and reported by clinicians as confusion or anxiety, as the current case attempts to illustrate.

The current case study, Ms A, is a brief psychodynamically oriented intervention for a patient with Luria's semantic aphasia. The aims are to illustrate the importance and relevance of applying our understanding of syntax problems in neurological rehabilitation; how deficits in syntax can influence patients' thoughts and behaviours; the limitations of cognitive assessment of receptive aphasia; the potential for countertransference to be applied as a complementary data source; the role receptive language has beyond language in sustaining reflexive consciousness; how these impairments compromise meaning-making and emotional adjustment in rehabilitation; and last, that incorporating these variables into case formulations can guide adjustments in technique in order to facilitate psychotherapeutic goals.

Case description

Neurological injury and sequelae

The patient, Ms. A, experienced a left lacunar infarct, as assessed by CT scan, and underwent a carotid endarterectomy. The precise location of the lacunes was not recorded. Lacunar strokes are defined as small subcortical infarcts (<15 mm in diameter) resulting from occlusion of a single perforating artery (Donnar, Norrving, Bamford, & Bogouslavsky, 2002). Lacunar stroke is also the most common manifestation of cerebral small-vessel disease (Micheli et al., 2008). A systematic review of 17 studies found cognitive impairment after lacunar stroke in the following domains: attention/working memory, executive functioning, memory, language and visuospatial function (Edwards, Jacova, Sepehry, Pratt, & Benavente, 2013); however, the language impairment in the review was not sub-divided into aphasia types.

Ms A was reported to have symptoms of relatively mild right-sided hemiplegia, language difficulties and some visual changes. She was quickly discharged home from acute care and initially received SLT outpatient support only. It was not until six months post-stroke that she was seen at the community neurological rehabilitation service outpatient clinic, where she received specialist neurological physiotherapy and occupational therapy. Her principal difficulty at that time was with activities of daily living, such as multi-tasking in the kitchen, and she received regular input from an experienced neurological occupational therapist. She was assessed by the occupational therapist to have "good verbal communication" and to have engaged well in these therapies.

Ms A was an Irish Catholic, one of five children raised in a farming community. At the time of the psychotherapeutic appointments, she was 62 years old. She had type 2 diabetes mellitus and was hypertensive. She reported a normal development and described a particular closeness to her paternal grandmother, who lived close by in the ancestral cottage. She described herself as a romantic, free-spirited child. Fantasy, faeries and stories were a feature of her childhood, and she drew upon fantasy and happy childhood memories through poetry at different points in her life. Aged 17, she became pregnant by a local boy. In 1970s Ireland, the Catholic church dominated the public discourse on morality and behaviour. It was common practice to send unmarried pregnant women and girls to stay with the Magdalene Sisters until the child was born. The children were then usually taken away from their mothers and given up for adoption. While staying with the Magdalene Sisters the women were essentially in servitude, carrying out long hours of menial work. A 2002 film *The Magdalene Sisters* portrayed life in the Magdalene Laundries in Dublin. So it was for Ms A who, at this moment of great vulnerability, was effectively banished into servitude with minimal contact with her family for seven months, until she carried the child to term. She experienced preeclampsia and was not permitted to hold or to see her child postpartum. She was told that her child lived for 16 hours postnatally and then died. She returned to Ireland many times over the years. During one of these trips, she searched for and was unable to locate birth or death certificates for her child.

Neither the time she spent away with the Magdalene Sisters nor the death of her baby were ever discussed openly in the family. On returning home, she quickly realised she could not stay. A few days after her return, she asked her grandmother for money to make the crossing to Liverpool and onwards to London. She arrived and was taken in by members of a local Irish community, who helped her to find her feet. Not long after arriving in London she met and married an English man, raising seven children and, in time, several grandchildren. She described her husband as an alcoholic and experienced physical and emotional abuse by him for many years. One day, after 24 years of marriage, following a particularly violent attack, she said she realised the abuse would never stop and decided to leave. With the support of a neighbour, she took the children still living at home to live for several months in a mobile home on the south coast of England. She later relocated to North London.

In terms of her pre-injury characteristics, she described herself as outgoing and a workaholic. She never had time to stop, or to dwell, never slowed down before her stroke. She appeared to fill her life with children and activity. She was an outreach worker at a children's centre for 20 years and fostered many children throughout her life. She also maintained a fascination and affection for faeries and had written many poems about them, mostly for her grandchildren. While not a hoarder, she reported her adult children would often criticise her for buying items that she did not need such as trinkets and ornaments for the house. At the time of her stroke, she had been in a 10-year relationship and was living with her partner and two of her adult children.

Neuropsychological assessment

During the initial contact with the community neurological rehabilitation service six months post-stroke, Ms A participated in cognitive screening using the Birmingham Cognitive Screen (BCoS; Humphreys, 2012). The BCoS is a broad screening tool which divides patients into impaired and unimpaired categories across many domains. Patients who score equal to or less than the fifth percentile compared with controls are considered to have an impairment. Ms A was assessed to be unimpaired in all aspects of the cognitive screen, except for immediate and delayed recall for auditory-verbal information, and visual extinction. Also during the initial contact with the community service, Ms A completed two mood questionnaires. She scored in the severe depression range on the Patient Health Questionnaire-9 (PHQ-9; Kroenke, Spitzer, & Williams, 2001) and in the moderately severe anxiety range on the Generalised Anxiety Disorder-7 scale (GAD-7; Spitzer, Kroenke, Williams, & Löwe, 2006). She expressed suicidal thoughts at that point but had no plan to act on these thoughts. A referral was made to community mental health services. She subsequently attended a six-week cognitive behavioural therapy (CBT) group for anxiety and depression with the mental health team; she reported this was helpful and that she no longer felt depressed.

Nine months post-stroke, there was a pattern of gradual disengagement from all therapies by the patient, including cancelled appointments and non-attendance. This was in the context of her long-term partner ending their relationship. He subsequently withdrew completely from contact. The persistence of the community occupational therapist resulted in follow-up assessments 10 months post-stroke. At that point, Ms A was re-assessed using the BCoS (Humphreys, 2012), and her immediate recall for verbal information was then assessed to be in the unimpaired range. She was in the moderately severe depression range on the PHQ-9, a slight improvement compared with assessment at six months; however, she also scored in the severe anxiety range on the GAD-7, a more severe level than at six months. The occupational therapist at that time also noted Ms A had become socially withdrawn.

Eleven months post-stroke, the patient was offered an appointment with the clinical psychologist at the community neurological rehabilitation service. She did not attend the first appointment and cancelled the second appointment because of feeling unwell. Ms A subsequently met the clinical psychologist for assessment. The patient reported difficulties with concentration and memory, and that she had lost control of her life and her emotions. The psychologist noted some difficulties in word-finding. She was referred to an acceptance and commitment therapy (ACT) group for neurological patients with a trainee clinical psychologist. She was also added to the waiting list for counselling at her GP practice and attended eight sessions with a counsellor. Eighteen months after her stroke, she was re-referred for community neurological rehabilitation by her GP for help with mild, residual right-sided weakness, visual problems, poor concentration and loss of confidence. Twenty-one months post-stroke, she attended four of six sessions of the ACT group. During a review appointment, Ms A indicated that she would like more support in adjusting to life after her stroke and the strong emotions she was experiencing, and was re-referred to clinical psychology.

Formulation

Twenty-three months post-stroke, Ms A presented for assessment with the therapist (AR). This was to be the first of only three formal psychotherapeutic appointments, each lasting 90 minutes. There was one subsequent face-to-face meeting, a system-level intervention in the context of the patient's benefits being withdrawn, and several telephone meetings. The therapeutic intervention was intensive short-term dynamic psychotherapy (ISTDP), though as we shall see, the focus of the three sessions was in removing barriers to engagement in psychotherapy. Ms A was well presented and had little problems with expressive language. She spoke fluently though quietly, with few hesitations and very occasional pauses to find a word. Her words and actions were appropriate and relevant to the situation; she spoke in a reasonably open way about her emotional difficulties. She was on the surface deferential, but the therapist also sensed a dogged determination. The therapist was also quickly struck by a note of desperation in her tone of voice, and he gained a sense of stuckness and helplessness in the patient. Ms A asked for the therapist's help understanding why she was so frequently tearful. Her speech was circumlocutory, and she frequently sought reassurance from the therapist, with variations of "Am I making sense?"

During the first appointment, the therapist experienced a mixture of countertransferential feelings. On the one hand, there was a sense of ancestral connection to the idyllic rural life Ms A described, of sharing in an innocent childhood experience of Ireland (she at times seemed better connected to that world than to her present reality). There were also resonances with the therapist's childhood as a devout Catholic, which mobilised a brief fantasy of healing the patient and the historic injustice enacted in the name of the church, perhaps healing his own wounds of lost faith in the process. On the other hand, there was also a countertransferential experience of ambiguous closeness with the patient – a somewhat surreal experience that the patient was being open about her suffering and was seeking emotional intimacy yet, despite a lot of seemingly appropriate words being exchanged, it felt that *meaning* was disappearing into an unfathomable chasm between therapist and patient. The therapist also experienced fleeting irritation; he sensed that he was not really being listened to. While the therapist sensed he was gaining some understanding of Ms A, it also seemed to him that Ms A was neither gaining much greater insight from opening up about her painful emotions, nor did he get the sense that she understood the therapist was building up such a picture.

The therapist began to consider the possibility that a neurological deficit was being encountered in the countertransference. He was curious about the aphasia and the patient's tendency to check if she was making sense to the therapist. Of course, checking in about making sense can occur for non-neurological reasons, for example, transferential feelings or projections onto the male therapist as a potential abuser, checking with the other as a defence against anxiety resulting from expected negative appraisal by the therapist, or habitually doubting one's reality. The patient confirmed her difficulty understanding language. She reported that she struggled to deeply process the meaning of spoken and written words: "I have to read things several times, over and over, so that it goes in, until I really get it – does that make sense?"

Drawing on Kaplan-Solms and Solms's conceptualisation of Mrs K, the therapist began to hypothesise that the patient's frequent question "Am I making sense" was indeed symptomatic of receptive aphasia; she was simply less able to monitor the content of *her own speech* reliably enough to be confident that she was making sense. In the context of not knowing whether what she had intended to say was actually what she had said, she became anxious that she had made a mistake and would appear foolish to the therapist. Consequently, she found it difficult to engage in conversation, both in terms of understanding and digesting language, but also being confident of her own words. It appeared that the combination of her relatively expressive fluency, her pleasant manner and good grasp of social cues had served to mask this subtle yet profound deficit, even from experienced clinicians. Indeed, both patient and therapist were experiencing, in parallel, an ambiguous closeness; of being in the presence of the other who wanted to engage in emotional intimacy, yet not being sure that their words or meanings were being fully understood. Both were wondering: "Am I making sense (to you)?"

Ms A presented with symptoms consistent with Luria's semantic aphasia, detected on the initial BCoS cognitive screen at six months as an impairment in working memory and delayed memory for auditory-verbal information and visuo-spatial difficulties. Notably, these ongoing deficits were not subsequently detected by the BCoS at 10 months. She was able to hear and understand individual words well and could speak fluently; however, she was experiencing a significant deficit in decoding auditory-verbal information according to the logico-grammatical rules of language. In other words, she had an impairment in her ability to understand the syntactical, grammatical relationships between words. This presented as a slowness to grasp the relationships between words or concepts, even with repeated exposure. Her problems with spatial orientation were also apparent and were detected on the initial BCoS at six months, another common symptom in semantic aphasia. For example, more than 2 years post-stroke she reported hanging a series of baskets upside down and making errors with a previously well-known knitting pattern, knitting some baubles inside-out.

The consequence for Ms A was that, because of her difficulties bringing the unconscious mental processes of the ego into conscious awareness through stabilised auditory-verbal associations, she was less able to engage in the therapeutic task of holding and synthesising the semantic content of the words she attached to her thoughts. In terms of her engagement in "normal mourning", this deficit contributed to her sense of being stuck, stuck in fog, in a word-soup, with limited ability to order meanings, to make sense of her reality, to move towards emotional catharsis in the context of her sadness and grief. There was also an overlap between her experience of semantic aphasia and her attempts to understand and process her losses since her stroke. She internally experienced this as being unable to make sense: "I can't make sense of it".

Psychotherapeutic intervention

The formulation highlighted to the therapist how easy it would be to engage in apparently meaningful but ultimately profoundly transient therapeutic interactions with the patient, with minimal impact on her understanding or feelings. The formulation allowed the therapist to avoid wasted effort by highlighting the importance of holding words stable in the patient's mind through repetition and writing. The patient was encouraged to bring a notebook to all subsequent sessions. In the second session, the patient wrote under the therapist's instruction: "I have receptive aphasia. This means that it is very difficult for me to understand the meaning of words. This means that I am often unsure if what I have said makes sense." She was encouraged to read the notes over repeatedly in session until, prioritising her subjective experience, she reported sensing the meaning had settled upon her, that she had been able to digest the meaning. In this way, the intervention served to stabilise the auditory-verbal traces, initially by using the therapist's auditory-verbal working memory and then through writing the words on a page.

Encouraging writing resonated with a past solution for processing emotions, writing poetry, to which the patient had returned to post stroke, and of course which held great potential for understanding and working through. The patient shared the content of the poems, which illustrated her struggles with semantic aphasia. Each poem is striking in the adherence to extremely short lines with minimal connections and linear, mono-thematic format. The description of trying to find "a way out of this maze, and back into my mind" in Poem 1 appears to capture her struggle with finding her way towards meaning, as if she could see the walls in front of her (words), but not the connection (syntax). Poem 2 appears to describe her difficulties in bringing the unconscious processes into conscious awareness: "I try to converse, With my own silly head" and also draws out the theme of confusion, while Poem 3 articulates her estrangement from herself: "I'm not the same person."

The therapeutic work ceased after Ms A received notice that her disability benefits were to be discontinued following a governmental assessment. She told the therapist that she could no longer afford the taxi journey. The therapist discussed the appeal process with Ms A and contributed a letter in support of the appeal, drawing specific attention to the subtle yet profound nature of her receptive aphasia. Her appeal was upheld.

Poem 1	*Poem 2*	*Poem 3*
Where is my life	Sitting here wondering	Damn this stroke
I don't quite know	Into the night	I hate it so
I've lost it somehow	When will this stroke	Everything is changed
Somewhere so	Ever be right	I'm not the same person
I sit and wait	I try to converse	Just the same name
And try to find	With my own silly head	It creeps up all a sudden
A way out of this maze	But all that comes out	And bites you on the bum
And back into my mind	Is mumbo jumbo instead	Then turns around
I know it's out there	To talk to myself	And runs away
But have I got it wrong	Really seems OK	And leaves you feeling numb
I've lost my words	But to say it out loud	My words all seem so muddled
But I've got to be strong	I'd rather not say	As I write and say
So stop the tears	Because some of my words	What seemed OK yesterday
And the senseless wait	They go into reverse	Is written wrong today
Just lift the latch	Causing confusion	It causes such confusion
And open the gate	It's really a curse	I don't know what to do
There's a world out there	Maybe the counselling	One day my plans are all there
You've got to find	Will help me in time	The next just hav'nt a clue
Open your eyes	If not I'll just settle	When will it get better
And open your mind.	To help me	That's what I want to know
	To be kind.	I feel such pain and again
		Just need to let it go

Results

The patient's grasp of the key technique of stabilising auditory-verbal information in mind through writing and re-reading, which resonated with past self-exploration through poetry, was the key achievement of the intervention. This enabled Ms A to understand crucial psychoeducational ideas about the nature of her aphasia and the impact it was having on her ability to make meaning. This supported more precise meaning-making and helped clarify her losses. Writing her thoughts, reading them over and over until the meaning settled in and new meanings emerged, enabled her to independently stay with and absorb their interconnected meanings. During a telephone review six months after the psychotherapy, she said: "I write everything down so I can explain it to myself. That is very helpful." Nonetheless, even with this key technique, it was clear that Ms A still could only partially process information and had ongoing difficulty with retention.

In terms of engaging in "normal mourning", it appeared to be more difficult for Ms A to come to terms with the changes since her stroke because of her problems with making meaning. The technique of writing and re-reading helped her to begin to make sense of her losses and sadness. She continued with this technique and made progress, albeit slowly. Approximately three years post injury, Ms A reported "I feel together with myself. I am alone now, but I like it. I sit in the garden, with my thoughts, writing poetry. I feel this is mental and emotional healing. I also think my memory is slowly improving." Lastly, the system-level intervention contributing a brief report in support of her benefit appeal was another success attributable to the formulation of her receptive aphasia.

Discussion

This brief psychodynamically oriented intervention applied Luria's concept of semantic aphasia to efficiently formulate a subtle yet profound receptive language deficit, which had been the major factor in the patient's reduced confidence about her ability to make sense to others, with emotional and behavioural consequences for her in terms of increased levels of anxiety, low mood, reduced confidence, reduced ability to engage in the process of normal mourning, withdrawal and social avoidance. This case highlights the importance of considering syntax problems in receptive aphasia and the impact this deficit can have on meaning-making and emotional processing. Ms A's receptive aphasia had clearly been underestimated or overlooked by several experienced clinicians, a testament to the subtlety of the deficit, or perhaps a reflection of the implicit assumption that receptive language ability does not have a role in other higher-order mental processes, such as reflexive consciousness. Her language deficits were suggested by the initial cognitive screening assessment (BCoS) six months post injury; however, the repeat cognitive screen and subsequent psychological assessment suggested her language abilities had mostly resolved by 10 months post injury. This case study suggests limitations of the classic cognitive assessment procedure in detecting subtle receptive aphasias.

Also highlighted by this case is the usefulness of countertransference as a data source in neuropsychological assessment as it was the countertransferential feeling of irritation that the therapist was not being listened to that led to questions and hypothesising about the presence of a deficit. The countertransference experienced fit with Lewis's (1999) type a – complementary feelings of frustration. It is possible that this was a feeling experienced by others in their relationships with Ms A. The countertransference facilitated the interpretation of apparent reassurance-seeking "Am I making sense?" into a formulation of receptive aphasia. In turn, the formulation directed the therapist to focus immediately on the hypothesised working memory deficit by supporting Ms A to understand and process key learning points by writing them in a notebook for re-reading and deeper processing, towards normal mourning.

Without the formulation, there were many junctures where the therapist might have incorrectly concluded that the patient was anxious and depressed because she had not come to terms with her losses because of her pre-morbid history, rather than correctly concluding she was anxious because she was struggling to make sense of her losses as a consequence of her neurological injury. In addition, the patient's frequently expressed *doubt* that she was making sense could very easily be misattributed to her anxiety, or to personality. The formulation also allowed the therapist to look beyond the receptive difficulties at the single-word level, to understand that there was a lack of structure to allow her to think about the relationships between things in time and space. Without checking for understanding, for deep processing, and without supporting the syntactic connections and resonances with other meanings, the therapeutic task was likely to be transient. It was perhaps for these reasons that the patient did not experience lasting benefit from CBT or ACT, with their reliance on auditory-verbal working memory and the top-down digestion of meaning.

The intervention employed a frequently used compensatory strategy – writing – as an essential adaptation to facilitate the beginnings of working through for Ms A. She required help to stabilise meaning in time and space, particularly the logico-grammatical rules and the syntactic structure, to establish connections in the relationships between things (Solms, 2013). It is noteworthy that Mrs K and Ms A's presentations were very similar: both were reality-orientated, with a sense of estrangement from the self and exhibited circumlocutory speech and word-finding difficulties. The key difference appeared to be in the reported subjective experience of gaps in consciousness: Mrs K reported this as a deficit more in keeping with the working-memory deficit hypothesis, whereas Ms A reported trying to find her way through a maze, through the connections between places, a problem not with the semantics, but with the syntax of language. Tentatively, this may capture the subjective differences in how acoustico-mnestic and semantic aphasias are experienced.

In addition to the limitations of single-case study design in terms of generalisability, the absence of a precise location of the lacunar infarcts and the potential presence of small-vessel disease were uncontrolled variables, which may have been factors in Ms A's presentation. The potentially diffuse effects associated with sub-cortical aphasia may indicate other sources of difficulty in organising meaning, such as dysexecutive problems. The very limited numbers of sessions meant there was little opportunity to explore how early life experiences and many years of domestic abuse had shaped Ms A's presentation, and additional sessions may also have allowed transferential and countertransferential feelings to develop.

Conclusions

This case study aimed to highlight the usefulness of Luria's concept of semantic aphasia in formulating and intervening in syntax problems in receptive aphasia, and adds support to the assertion that countertransference can be a useful data source in neuropsychological assessment and psychotherapy with neurological patients, and can assist in uncovering subtle deficits. Detecting the deficit pointed to the key adaptation required – writing and re-reading to compensate for the receptive language deficit, supporting reflexive consciousness and thereby helping the patient to engage in the task of psychotherapy towards normal mourning and working through. This can also be conceptualised as helping the patient with self-talk, as set out in Figure 2.2. The patient's unstable syntactic structure was the

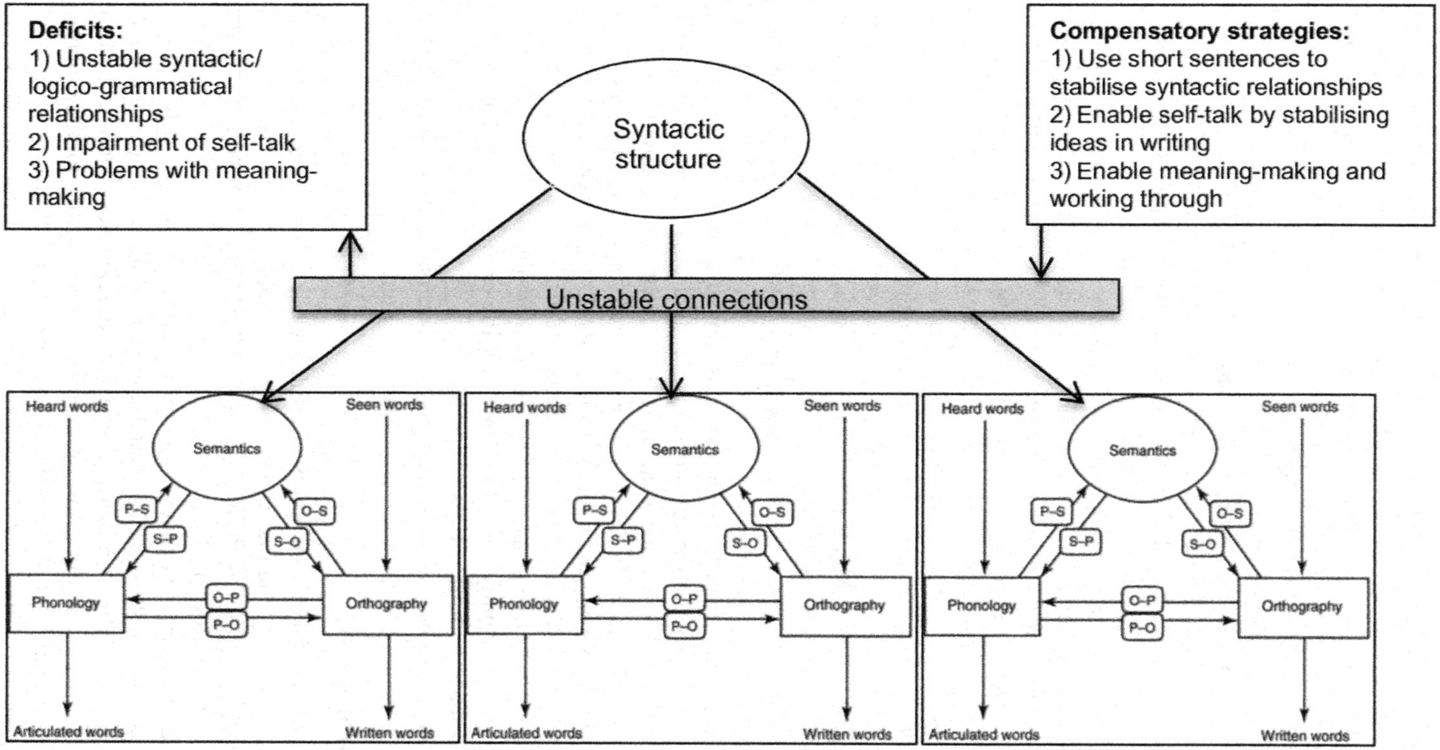

Figure 2.2 Syntactic model using the cognitive model of single-word processing

Source: Adapted from Patterson & Shewell, 1987

key area of deficit, suggesting simple compensatory strategies. While the patient was able to understand that she had had a stroke, she was experiencing real-world consequences of her semantic aphasia; she doubted that she was making sense, felt her sense of identity was undermined and experienced high levels of anxiety, low confidence and low mood. The compensatory strategy of writing and re-reading to stabilise the connections among semantic contents, which luckily resonated with her own experiences of writing poetry, helped her to move towards normal mourning.

In addition to the implications for the patient's processes, there are also implications for professionals in terms of how easy it is to overlook this relatively subtle deficit. In the UK context, it appears that the focus of assessment in receptive aphasia is often slanted towards understanding ability with single words, with less focus on patients' abilities to synthesise meaning. This suggests that, for some patients, there may be opportunities to engage in slow structured work to help deeply process meaning, with a focus on syntax with potentially great benefit for the patient's emotional adjustment.

Future directions

At least two conceptual questions arising from this case study may warrant more investigation: First, is the confusion and anxiety often seen in receptive aphasia due to problems in reflexive consciousness, and does this typically result in problems in meaning-making and therefore present a barrier normal mourning? And second, in semantic aphasia, is such confusion and anxiety due to the loss of ability to make connections between semantic ideas? To answer these questions, patients with receptive aphasia could be routinely assessed for the kind of syntactic deficits presented in both the current case and Mrs K, towards the development of potentially novel rehabilitation strategies.

References

Bishop, D. V. (1989). *Test for the reception of grammar: (TROG)*. London: Medical Research Council.

Caplan, D., Hildebrandt, N., & Marshall, J. C. (1988). *Disorders of syntactic comprehension*. Cambridge, MA: MIT Press.

Doesborgh, S. (2004). *Assessment and treatment of linguistic deficits in aphasic patients*. Doctoral dissertation, University Medical Center Rotterdam, Erasmus, MC.

Donnar, G. A., Norrving, B., Bamford, J. M., & Bogouslavsky, J. (2002). Classification of subcortical infarcts. In *Subcortical stroke* (pp. 27–34). Oxford: Oxford Medical Publications.

Edwards, J. D., Jacova, C., Sepehry, A. A., Pratt, B., & Benavente, O. R. (2013). A quantitative systematic review of domain-specific cognitive impairment in lacunar stroke. *Neurology*, *80*(3), 315–322.

Francis, D. R., Clark, N., & Humphreys, G. W. (2003). The treatment of an auditory working memory deficit and the implications for sentence comprehension abilities in mild "receptive" aphasia. *Aphasiology*, *17*(8), 723–750.

Freud, S. (1923b). *The ego and the Id* (Standard ed., Vol. XIX). London: Hogarth.

Horan, J. J. (2016). *A systematic review of aphasia therapy outcomes research.* Doctoral dissertation, Cleveland State University.

Howard, D., & Patterson, K. E. (1992). *The pyramids and palm trees test: A test of semantic access from words and pictures.* Bury St. Edmunds, Suffolk: Thames Valley Test Company.

Humphreys, G. (2012). *Birmingham cognitive screen.* London: Taylor & Francis.

Kaplan-Solms, K., & Solms, M. (2000). *Clinical studies in neuro-psychoanalysis.* London: Karnac Books.

Kay, J., Lesser, R., & Coltheart, M. (1992). *Psycholinguistic Assessments of Language Processing in Aphasia (PALPA).* Hove, East Sussex: Lawrence Erlbaum Associates.

Kroenke, K., Spitzer, R., & Williams, J. (2001). The PHQ-9: Validity of a brief depression severity measure. *Journal of General Internal Medicine, 16*, 606–613.

LaPointe, L. (2005). *Aphasia and related neurogenic language disorders* (3rd ed.). New York: Thieme.

Lewis, L. (1999). Transference and countertransference in psychotherapy with adults having traumatic brain injury. In *Psychotherapeutic interventions for adults with brain injury or stroke: A clinician's treatment resource* (pp. 113–130). Madison, CT: Psychological Press.

Luria, A. R. (1963). *Restoration of function after brain injury.* Oxford: Macmillan.

Micheli, S., Agnelli, G., Palmerini, F., Caso, V., Venti, M., Alberti, A. . . . Paciaroni, M. (2008). Need for extensive diagnostic work-up for patients with lacunar stroke. *Journal of Neurology, 255*(5), 637–642.

Moore, P. A., Salas, C. E., Dockree, S., & Turnbull, O. H. (2017). Observations on working psychoanalytically with a profoundly amnesic patient. *Frontiers in Psychology, 8*, 1418.

Patterson, K., & Shewell, C. (1987). Speak and spell: Dissociations and word class effects. In M. Coltheart, G. Sartori, & R. Job (Eds.), *The cognitive neuropsychology of language* (pp. 273–294). London: Erlbaum.

Pinker, S. (1994). *The language instinct: How the mind creates language.* London, UK: Penguin Books.

Prigatano, G. P., Borgaro, S., & Caples, H. (2003). Non-pharmacological management of psychiatric disturbances after traumatic brain injury. *International Review of Psychiatry, 15*(4), 371–379.

Salas, C. E., & Coetzer, R. (2015). Is concreteness the invisible link between altered emotional processing, impaired awareness and mourning difficulties after traumatic brain injury? *Neuropsychoanalysis, 17*(1), 3–18.

Salis, C., Hwang, F., Howard, D., & Lallini, N. (2017, February). Short-term and working memory treatments for improving sentence comprehension in aphasia: A review and a replication study. In *Seminars in speech and language* (Vol. 38, No. 01, pp. 29–39). New York: Thieme Medical Publishers.

Solms, M. (2013). The conscious Id. *Neuropsychoanalysis, 15*(1), 5–19.

Spitzer, R. L., Kroenke, K., Williams, J. B., & Löwe, B. (2006). A brief measure for assessing generalized anxiety disorder: The GAD-7. *Archives of Internal Medicine, 166*(10), 1092–1097.

Whitworth, A., Webster, J., & Howard, D. (2005). *A cognitive neuropsychological approach to assessment and intervention in aphasia: A clinician's guide.* New York: Psychology Press.

Chapter 3

A personal construct psychology approach to aphasia

Cathy Sparkes

Introduction

Aphasia is a language disorder which typically occurs after a stroke – it affects the production and/or comprehension of speech, the ability to read and/or write. Parr, Byng, Gilpin, and Ireland (1997) reminds us that 'language is the currency of relationships . . . aphasia reduces the influence of one person in what was once a two-way process'. Parr goes on to reflect that 'Aphasia does not just affect those who have it. The impact of language impairment is felt across entire social networks, by partners, children, parents, siblings, friends and colleagues.' Aphasia can affect all aspects of an individual's life and a person's identity. Working with someone whose language is compromised in this way takes commitment and creativity by both the client and the practitioner.

The aim of this article is to provide insight into how a personal construct psychology (PCP) approach has helped one woman with aphasia to work with her counsellor to make sense of her new situation. The series of sessions illustrates the approach to counselling I offer clients who have communication difficulties and who need creative ways to support the development of a personal meaning in their new life. I hope that by reading through this case, the approach taken will illuminate how PCP can provide a foundation for working in this way with people with communication difficulties.

I start by describing PCP, consider how PCP relates to communication difficulties, introduce those involved in the therapy (Cathy and Ruth), give an account of therapy interactions and offer some reflections and learning points.

What is personal construct psychology?

The theory of PCP is not only a counselling theory, but also a theory which relates to everyone, to help each of us understand how an individual construes (understands and interacts with) the world. George Kelly, who developed PCP, set out three key foundations: constructive alternativism, person as scientist and reflexivity (Kelly, 1955).

Constructive alternativism

This is Kelly's philosophy which suggests that as individuals we are continually trying to grasp the real world by constructing our own version of it, and trying to anticipate an event or situation. To achieve this, each person develops their own set of constructs. A construct is an abstraction – we abstract our own personal meaning from the world we interact with. We make bi-polar discriminations of similarities and differences between elements, that is, people, objects, events. The nature of the relationship between the two poles of a construct is one of contrast, for example, when an individual makes sense of something in a certain way, that person is implicitly saying what it is not. For example, someone might construe the contrast to 'driven' as 'lazy', but someone else might construe the contrast to 'driven' as 'spontaneous'. It is important to say that the words we use to describe our constructs are merely verbal labels. Many constructs we have may not even have words to describe them, and these may be very core to us. We construe by thinking and also by feeling, looking, listening, touching, tasting and moving. PCP therapy focusses on understanding how each client construes the world and to what extent this serves them well or not.

Person as scientist

Kelly (1955) proposes we are all in our own particular way scientists. Behaviour is seen as an experiment to test out our theory of the world. Peggy Dalton explains that in therapy, 'The two people involved are seen as scientists, each contributing in partnership, to experiments for change. Each has his or her particular expertise. The client has all the 'data', the material from which some resolutions of difficulty may be made. The counsellor has experience in exploring such material and helping the client to make something new out of it' (Dalton, 1994, p. 22). As scientists together, the therapist and client work collaboratively to try to move the client's construing forward.

Reflexivity

PCP is a theory that applies to all of us. The notion of reflexivity proposes that I as an individual and as a counsellor have to understand how the theory can and does apply to me as much as it applies to each person I work with. I need to be aware of how my constructs are organised and equally I need to listen to and subsume (step into the shoes of) my client and their construing. I know my own constructs in my role as an independent PCP counsellor include, for instance:

- Process connected rather than outcome driven
- Person-informed rather than system-led
- Shaped by regular reviews rather than fixed to a pre-determined specific number of sessions

- Open and transparent rather than shrouded in mystery
- Context-related (outward-facing) rather than restricted to the therapy room
- Innovative and experimental rather than rigid and stagnant

In addition to my own and my client's personal constructs, there are also professional constructs. These are the ways in which a practitioner refers to the client's construing of their world. Kelly (1955) says that professional constructs are 'avenues of movement as seen by the therapist (counsellor) just as the client's personal constructs are potential avenues of movement as seen by the client' (Kelly, 1955). These professional constructs refer to how or why a client might or might not be moving psychologically. An example of this is the construct of tightening or loosening. This relates to how someone may be holding onto an existing way of construing (tight) rather than experimenting with alternative, more varying predictions (loose). The professional constructs help me to determine the ebb and flow of a client's construing and ultimately assist them in moving forward.

'Personal construct psychotherapy does not have a strict recipe of actions to follow, because it is personally directed' (Dalton, 2005). PCP does not provide a set of instructions; there are no 'norms' or pre-determined expectations. Instead, this approach requires the practitioner to collaborate with a client moment by moment. Kelly (1955) states: 'We take the stand that there are always some alternative constructions available to choose among in dealing with the world. No one needs paint himself [sic] into a corner, no one needs to be completely hemmed in by circumstances; no one needs to be a victim of their biography'. Both the client and the therapist have multiple options for how they work together.

PCP, brain injury and communication difficulties

In 1972, Fay Fransella first introduced personal construct psychology into the world of therapy with people with communication difficulties, in the field of stammering. Peggy Dalton, SLT and psychotherapist, also worked in this area and recognised the relevance and applicability of such a theory in related specialties. Dalton applied PCP not only to working with people with brain injury, but also notably applied it to her own personal situation. She describes the experience of living with her husband, who had himself experienced a neurological event with resulting severe memory loss. Her recognition that PCP supported and guided her in this personal journey is clear and highlights the relevance of PCP to everyone (Dalton, 1990).

When a new situation arises for an individual, such as a stroke, that person's own unique construct system is affected in some way. 'Where brain damage causes loss of perception, loss of language, loss of memory, for example, the person not only has a new situation to make sense of but is less equipped to re-organise his or her construing' (Dalton, 2005). An individual will try to make sense of and look for meaning in their new situation using the constructs which are available to them. But that person may need to re-organise their construing or re-construe themselves and the world around them. 'Kelly describes counselling as a "situation in which one person helps another achieve a psychological reconstruction of life. Thus, the aim of counselling is to open up the personal world of experience in which the person feels stuck so they may find alternative ways of coping with the world of events which confronts them"'(Jones, 1988).

Dalton (1994) says that a counsellor's first priority in relation to their clients 'is to help them to clarify what is troubling them in the context of their experience of life as a whole'. Dalton (1994) notes that 'severe communication problems may preclude the use of some procedures and demand imaginative modification in the use of others' and suggests a range of creative, non-verbal materials, for example, pictures, the use of drawings, music, in order to access someone's constructs.

Case study: Cathy and Ruth

Cathy: PCP counsellor

I work as a PCP counsellor with individuals, couples and family groups, in independent practice. I specialise in supporting people with neurological conditions who are living with communication and/or cognitive difficulties. I worked previously as a speech and language therapist (SLT) in this clinical field, in the NHS, for 19 years. I carry that knowledge and experience into my current roles and relationships. My counselling practice centres on PCP, and this approach allows my experiences through my professional and personal life to influence how I work with clients, families and colleagues.

In my practice, I receive referrals for individuals at a time in their rehabilitation where they have received some or all of a range of therapies but progress has typically started to slow. This timing often dovetails with a need for them to reach out and access a space to consider their new self as a whole as they prepare to move forward. I work with people whose purpose often includes an attempt to understand who they are now, recognise who they can turn to for what and understand how to live in a meaningful way, following their injury or diagnosis.

My approach is centred on the importance for each individual to have the freedom to work in their own style, and at their own pace, towards their own hoped-for direction. I recognise the value of goals, outcomes and structures. Working with someone is a constant juggle of timing, content and rhythm determined by the alliance of me as the therapist, the client and the dynamic of the relationship. One essential element is the need to be transparent with theory and practice as applied in all sessions. I bear in mind the importance of the two experts (i.e. both my client and me) in the room. So I often refer to my background, experiences, values and styles when discussing or reflecting on counselling options with my clients. At the same time, I actively seek possibilities for the client to share their skills and knowledge.

My purpose is to enter a dialogue with each individual in which I attempt to grasp their perspectives, help them untangle the complexity of their life and make sense of the choices available to them. When I first started working with people as an SLT, I often used the analogy of the client as the driver and me in the passenger seat. Now, as a PCP counsellor, I prefer to use the analogy of learner driver (client) and driving instructor (therapist) in a vehicle with dual controls. We share the driving and navigating. An individual may have a vision of where they want to go or a potential destination, but possibly no equivalent of a steering wheel, gears or satellite navigation system.

When working with someone who finds it a challenge to communicate their own views and perspectives, wants and needs, aspirations and dreams, both the client and I need to acknowledge that our work together will be multi-faceted. I enjoy developing and using a wide variety of styles, approaches and imaginative bespoke tools and techniques. Throughout the introductory and subsequent counselling sessions, I regularly use a visual record. This typically starts with a blank sheet of paper which the client and I can use as a focus. We may use several sheets, which can include drawings, written words and symbols often in the style of mind maps, which are a way to visually organise the information both the client and I express. There is a central theme or topic, and ideas branch out from that. These sheets provide an ongoing and shared reference point during sessions, at the end of a session and as a summary tool at the completion of a series of sessions. I start by opening up a discussion in whatever way possible regarding the client's communication to determine how to facilitate and support our interactions. By modelling a variety of ways to communicate, showing openness in experimenting and a keenness to listen to a client's viewpoints, we can start to establish a shared notion of how we might work together.

My introductory session with someone is an opportunity to see the chemistry or the 'fit' between myself and a client; introducing who I am and offering someone the chance to express what they can about themselves. I share my professional experiences and background and explain that my approach is innovative and evolving. I may also reference some of my own constructs to clarify not only how I can work but also the ways or styles I prefer not to embrace. I bring into the working space materials which help each individual to understand and recognise that I am open to working creatively with them. The emphasis is on how we can strive to find our way through the challenges together.

My role as a PCP counsellor is to understand the interconnected and hierarchical web of constructs and construing which an individual uses to support the meaning they make of life in its new form. In this way I can begin to understand not only their present situation but possible future options. Each individual is a scientist, whatever their skills or problems, and I construe them as the expert in themselves learning about their own construing and how to re-construe life. I enter the room with my own set of constructs and expectations and will be met by the constructs and expectations of the client and often those of their family and friends too. My intent is to suspend my own personal construing and create an environment where we can learn from each other about what and how we both can contribute to our collaboration ahead of us.

My aims with Ruth have included understanding how she construes herself and her close family now and helping Ruth consider the alternative ways to construe herself and her world differently, which in turn may help her achieve her goals of interacting more meaningfully with family and friends.

Ruth: client

Ruth is a 65-year-old family-focussed woman who is a mother, partner, sister, grandmother and friend. Ruth was always (according to her partner and son) the 'go-to person' when anyone needed help. She worked as a jewellery designer but is now retired. Ruth enjoyed creative arts, in particular films and music. She lives with her partner (John) and two live-in carers (Sarah and Jen, who are long-standing friends). Ruth has a son (Marcus), a daughter (Emma) and one grandson (Joshua). She spoke three languages in addition to English before her stroke.

Ruth was referred to me by an SLT (Caroline), because they both felt that Ruth was at a point where she was reluctant to use alternative communication approaches given the absence of useful speech. She was, as a result, starting to withdraw from her family and friends' networks. Caroline hoped that if Ruth worked with a specialist counsellor, Ruth might reach a point where she would feel more comfortable engaging with others in spite of her communication difficulties and potentially feel more at ease to try some alternative means of interacting.

Following Ruth's stroke, she received three months of inpatient rehabilitation and at home has received and continues to receive occupational therapy, physiotherapy and speech and language therapy (although she decided to take a break from this once I became involved). Ruth experiences moderate aphasia – her comprehension is sufficient for everyday conversation when well supported – and severe expressive aphasia. Ruth can understand single written words and short concrete sentences; she cannot use writing in a useful way to communicate. Ruth communicates through 'total communication': gesture, facial expression, pointing and body language. Ruth is able to make some choices when offered materials with which to communicate. She has a reliable yes/no response when asked simple, concrete questions.

Ruth now has a different role in the family and is dependent on her family, carers and friends for many activities. Ruth spends much of her time in a wheelchair at home, can walk with a stick with the help of one person and needs help with personal and domestic care. She goes out with her partner on occasion to art galleries, coffee shops and the cinema. Ruth has indicated via the use of gesture and responses to yes/no questions that she would like to have more choice in her activities, increase the frequency of such trips and widen her social opportunities in the future. She frequently indicated through pointing to her mouth and vocalising frustration, that her lack of speech is the reason she cannot go out.

Therapy together: Cathy and Ruth

'Personal construct counselling is more to do with approaching a client with a particular frame of mind than with specific theoretical details about what one should do and specific techniques to use' (Fransella & Dalton, 1990).

Ruth and I started to work together 20 months after her stroke, for a total of eight sessions over a seven-month period. Following an introductory session, the therapeutic intervention evolved where the format of each subsequent session was configured and agreed by Ruth and Cathy at the preceding one.

Even from the first session with Ruth, I could see that despite her difficulties, she was attentive and interested as opposed to passive and disengaged (my constructs), leading to a sense of optimism (shown by Ruth's smiling and stroking my hand) on both sides about our future work together. Throughout our time, she has shown an enthusiasm to try new and different ways to work towards the goal of reconnecting with her life and her world. I was there to help support her in re-gaining some control, connection and confidence with key people in her life.

Throughout our sessions, I demonstrated my respect for Ruth being an 'expert' in herself. I used this approach from the outset, ensuring that Ruth was able to express her views, ideas and thoughts and ensuring that my communication style enabled this. I took time to build a rapport with Ruth in order to give her space and a 'voice'. Throughout the sessions I regularly spoke about and elaborated through drawings, our relationship as an evolving collaborative team. I was keen to listen to her story and share my professional story with Ruth too so she could appreciate the knowledge and skills I brought into the room. I explained that I was helping her to help me to help her as if we were co-explorers. I was offering her a way we could work together, but one that incorporated her own style and personality.

In this role relationship we developed a deep respect for each other, through both non-verbal and verbal avenues. I opened up meaningful and real conversations with Ruth to help her look at her own life now, how her life was before her stroke and as it could be in the future. I explained how PCP counselling was centred on us working alongside each other. I listened to her wishes and aspirations and she to mine. We have not been tied to a specific route or target; we are designing our map together as we move from session to session – as travellers both setting out in our roles as scientists and experimenting with our work together.

PCP sees all behaviour as an experiment, and this means that counselling is based on enquiry rather than interpretation. The client is responsible for choosing the experiments in their role of scientist. Each individual client holds the answers to their own future. The counsellor's job is to help to pinpoint what those answers might be.

The therapy story

Sessions one to three

At the introductory session, Ruth and I made a tentative plan for our work together. I explained that we could experiment as we moved forward with how the sessions might transpire and that we would review this aspect regularly. We agreed three further sessions after the introductory session and then a review session with John and Marcus. I made it clear that we would be checking in with each other at the end of each session, in case a different style or direction might be more useful.

Session one: Ruth and Cathy

As I approached our introductory session together, I knew that there had been huge changes and challenges for Ruth since her stroke. I found this information from a report from and conversation with the SLT, and a phone call with Ruth's son. I anticipated that she was now in a position where she had to reconstrue herself from being a highly communicative, articulate woman to someone who sees herself as severely restricted and isolated by her communication disabilities. Her stroke and aphasia were likely to be affecting her relationships with her partner, family and friends, and they too would have to be reconstruing her in her new role.

At the first session with Ruth, my starting place was a blank canvas, a plain sheet of paper which I often refer to as a 'possibility space'. During this session, we introduced ourselves and started to get to know each other. Ruth used gesture and facial expression, and I used verbal language but also gesture and facial expression too. In this way, Ruth started to relax (as evidenced by her facial expression and body language) and engaged in the therapy process. I recorded what I was discovering about Ruth on the blank sheets of paper, using drawing and writing; she was able to see everything I produced. I was keen to show Ruth that it was important to me to start to understand how she construes her new world. I showed Ruth the materials I had brought with me which I felt might support our conversation, and I invited her to show me objects in or around the space we were in, which could be used as a tangible way to communicate with me about her life.

My materials and resources included:

- Paper and pens: plain paper, felt-tip pens, blank cards, Post-it notes
- Pictures: postcards, picture cards, photos from magazines, internet images, Evoke cards (2009)
- Three-dimensional objects: buttons, shells, stones
- Copies of drawings: 'Blob Books' (Wilson & Long, 2008), 'Drawing on your emotions' (Sunderland & Engleheart, 2015)

Together we noticed what was in and around the room in her house, including:

- A calendar
- The garden, including a cat
- A wide variety of DVDs
- Photos in frames
- Jewellery in boxes
- A variety of 'total communication' resources from the SLT, including a communication chart, SLT picture cards

Through sharing with each other all the alternative materials we could use in therapy, Ruth could see that we were forming a tight-knit pair. We could each use any items from our own or each other's set of resources in our future sessions together and in this way start to experiment with new ideas and concepts.

Session two: Ruth and Cathy

As for many therapy sessions, I came to this session with a loose plan to enable Ruth to talk about life before and after her stroke, perhaps focussing on people in her family and friends network. I offered this as a starting point and reflected back to the first session, reminding Ruth that we could use any/all of our joint materials. When I had first arrived for the session, Ruth had noticed an unusual ring I was wearing. She indicated, using facial expression, gesture and pointing that she used to work as a jewellery maker and designer. I suggested we might explore the family/friends connections and invited her to use any of our joint materials. Ruth indicated by pointing to her carer to access the jewellery boxes and that she would like to use some of her own jewellery for this session. Ruth's initiation of accessing the jewellery was an example of her understanding of what our sessions could be – she was aware that she had choices in the materials we used and that she could take control in this way.

I asked Ruth to think of key people in her life (this could be family or friends) and then to choose an item of jewellery to represent each person. In this way there was a very concrete and clear way for Ruth to communicate her perspectives on these people. The people she chose, via her communication photo book, were: John, Marcus, Emma, Sarah, Jen and herself. I witnessed Ruth considering carefully each piece of jewellery she selected. I was available to support Ruth, but she was focussed on the process and engrossed in delving into her box of jewellery. I used a blank sheet of paper on which Ruth could place each piece of jewellery. As she made her selections by pointing to the photo book, Ruth indicated whom the jewellery was representing, and I wrote that name on the sheet. By the end of the process, each person was represented on the page.

Once Ruth had assigned an item of jewellery to each person, I was open to moving forward with a discussion around how she construed each person. But Ruth indicated by tapping my arm, pointing and nodding, that she was enjoying working with the jewellery and asked to continue with this approach. So, I suggested that we use some alternative pieces of jewellery to look at her timeline: before the stroke, now and in the future. Ruth agreed this was a good idea, through nodding. She chose some different pieces of jewellery from her boxes for each time period first and then was keen to communicate about her selections. Through interacting with Ruth, offering a range of spoken choices supported by written words, around what each selection might mean for Ruth, we developed a few words for each item elaborating the meaning of each choice. I checked with Ruth at each point and at the end that she was in agreement with my selection of 'verbal labels' which I noted on the sheet (Figure 3.1).

Before stroke: Love, lots of parts, strong, committed, easy going
Now: Vulnerable, small pieces, delicate, fragmented
The future: Connected, want to feel stronger

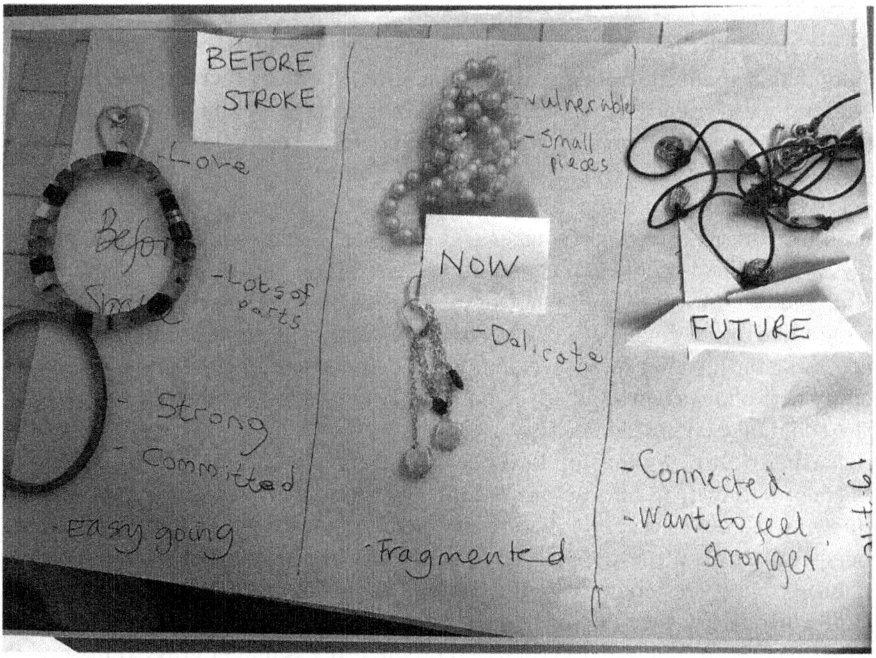

Figure 3.1 Before the stroke, now and the future

I observed and shared with Ruth that I noticed that a key theme – 'strong' – was emerging through this session. When I see a recurring word, idea or theme I will share this with a client as this might suggest that it is a core or important construct for that person. However, how Ruth now sees 'strong' may be different from before her stroke. This was something for us both to investigate in another session.

Session three: Ruth and Cathy

At the start of the session, I showed Ruth the sheet (see Figure 3.1) to remind her of the conversation we had had during the previous session. Ruth indicated through gesturing 'stronger' using a flexed arm and pointing to the phrase 'want to feel stronger' that she was keen to look more specifically in this session at what this meant to her. This time she indicated through pointing at my basket of resources that she wanted to use something from there, and I offered her some photos from current magazines of people in the news (royalty, politicians and celebrities). On one sheet of paper, I wrote the word 'strong', said the word and also indicated the meaning through flexing my own arm, as Ruth had done on several occasions. On another sheet of paper, I wrote a selection of verbal labels, referring to each with the relevant spoken word, which Ruth could choose from for the contrast to 'strong', including tired, weak, nervous, gentle, frail and soft. The aim was for both of us to understand both ends of the construct. By understanding the contrast to 'strong', it would help us both to assign more detailed meaning to 'strong'. Ruth chose 'weak', by pointing to that specific word and nodding as I said the word too.

I asked Ruth to differentiate which people in the photos she thought were 'strong' rather than the contrast 'weak', through placing the magazine photos accordingly. I asked her which she would prefer to be. Ruth indicated by pointing she would prefer to be 'strong'. But how did Ruth see this? The following is an extract of this conversation in which total communication was being used by both of us, in particular drawing and writing (me), gesture and facial expression (both of us):

CATHY: 'Why is being strong important?'
RUTH: Pointed first to the sheet (see Figure 3.1) where the word 'connected' is written and then moving her finger between the two of us for (as I understood it) being connected.
CATHY: 'Strong means connected?'
RUTH: Nodded
CATHY: 'How would you know that someone was 'strong'?'
RUTH: Used a combination of eye pointing, facial expression and responses to my yes/no questions and non-verbal communication, leading to the agreed spoken and written verbal labels:

- Positive in life
- Trying new activities
- Dipping a toe
- Pushing boundaries
- Physically strong

CATHY: 'How would you know that someone was 'weak'?'
RUTH: Used a combination of methods of communicating as before, resulting in these ascribed jointly agreed verbal labels:

- Giving up
- Standing still
- No get up and go
- Not where I want to be

Ruth communicated very clearly regarding her statement of 'I want to feel stronger', expressing this again by flexing her bicep. A further conversation developed over how connected Ruth feels with those around her, distinguishing between different people in her network. I asked Ruth how she can and does connect with people (referencing her photo book), and she indicated by pointing to items in her room: music, TV, films, shared activities and conversations.

Reflecting at the end of this session and on the process, we communicated with each other about how Ruth might become stronger and increase her connections with people: recognising who to depend on and for what, how to try new activities and go out more often. By way of a summary, I divided a blank page in two, and I wrote my understanding of Ruth's views of 'strong' and 'weak', saying each word or phrase aloud to ensure I had represented Ruth's views correctly:

- 'Strong': aim to enjoy life, try new things, experiment, speech not good, communication OK
- 'Weak': don't go out much, stay at home, feels sorry for self, sad, hiding and crying, speech not good, communication not good

Through these first three dynamic and creative sessions together, we found out that Ruth wants to be 'stronger'. For Ruth, this means being connected with her key people, trying activities (old and new) and starting to experiment with life. We pursued this theme at the start of our next session.

Sessions four and five

As part of PCP's professional constructs – ways for the practitioner to describe how the client is seeing the world – there are various cycles of construing. One of these is the CPC cycle which refers to Circumspection, Pre-emption and Control. This is a flexible framework for making decisions at numerous levels, from the overarching purpose of therapy through to the detail of an interaction. It is how I open up conversations about how to plan interventions and how I challenge where we might be going or suggest a change of direction.

The CPC cycle comprises:

1 *Circumspection:*
This is the phase where we look at what options are available. I present some choices but offer a client the chance to bring some to the table too. This could be seen as a brainstorming stage where all contributions remain valid.
2 *Pre-emption:*
This is the stage where the multiple contributions we both bring are reduced to a critical issue on which a choice could be made – typically a choice of two contrasting options.
3 *Control:*
This is the point at which the client and I are able to take the preferred choice forward – the one which has most meaning and/or offers the greatest possibilities for elaboration and translation into an action.

Session four: Ruth and Cathy

This session was the opportunity for a review of how we had been working together, in preparation for a session with John and Marcus. To be ready to discuss how the subsequent sessions might be configured, Ruth and I created a mind map together in which we shared everything we had worked on (the central theme). This initial loosening of ideas was an opportunity for us to share our perspectives. We agreed that this would form the basis of discussions with John and Marcus. Ruth made it clear to me that she wanted to share with them the overall work we had done so far, but she did not want to share our more detailed work. She expressed this by pointing to her mouth as if 'shhh' and then pointing to some of the sheets we had worked on previously.

Once Ruth and I had created this initial mind map, we then agreed to make the information more explicit. Ruth and I used Post-it notes to highlight the key themes we had explored. This whole process was part of the *circumspection phase* of the CPC cycle. Together we had identified five meaningful areas which Ruth considered as options to focus on in the next phase of our work together, but we also agreed that we needed to distil this to one or two. I explained that rather than five areas (shown by my counting on my fingers), it would be important to narrow down to one or two, so that sessions could be more focussed.

Session five: Ruth, John, Marcus and Cathy

Having Ruth with her partner, John, and son, Marcus, in the room created a new dynamic for this session. I took the lead, with Ruth's nod for me to do so. I started the session by sharing the mind map sheet that Ruth and I had created at the previous session in order to facilitate a discussion around the key choices to work from.

The purpose of the session was to consider the five areas and use these as a springboard for how to move forward:

- Relationships
- What makes Ruth happy
- Feeling stronger
- Feelings
- Before stroke, now and future

The visual representation of Ruth's views was a really important part of her 'voice' whilst in the room with the four of us. John and Marcus also shared their views regarding how they viewed the sessions and the benefits as they saw them.

As the conversation moved forward, the two areas Ruth, and therefore we, kept returning to were: 'Feeling stronger' and 'Relationships', with Ruth pointing to these emphatically. This was the *pre-emption phase* of the CPC cycle. As these two areas were being highlighted, I offered them to Ruth as a way of helping us to determine the next phase. Interestingly, as is often the case with therapy, the 'goal posts' changed. Ruth indicated that she wanted to work on both (I realise they are not mutually exclusive) and that the choice of how to progress was more related to who might work together on each one. Ruth used pointing to people in the room very effectively to communicate this view. We returned to the circumspection phase and opened out the choices regarding combinations of people who could be involved and styles of approach. The communal suggestions included:

- A combination of people (family and friends) in one-to-one, pair and group scenarios;
- Intervention and review opportunities; and
- Options around ending counselling.

Through additional conversations we came down to two key possibilities – either one-to-one work with Ruth and me or couples work with Ruth, John and me. So we had moved to the pre-emption phase once again – the choice of two. Throughout the whole of this process, Ruth remained at the centre of the decision making. Ruth then indicated through pointing and facial expression that she wanted to 'experiment' by convening a session with her, John and me together. This represented the *control phase.* I was incredibly pleased with how Ruth made this decision as she was demonstrating not only her understanding of the value of experimentation but was also 'dipping her toe' in a new way of working and being, which was one way she saw as 'being stronger'. Everyone agreed with this plan and so session six was with Ruth and John together. The therapy path had been renegotiated.

Sessions six to eight

Session six: Ruth, John and Cathy

In this first session with Ruth and John together, I suggested that we communicate about the possibilities for this session and beyond. We agreed that the purpose was to provide a mechanism through which John could learn about the importance and value of Ruth having enough space to share her perspectives. We linked this with a conversation at a previous session when Ruth communicated that she does not get the chance to express herself at mealtimes. This session and additional sessions could be the opportunity for John to witness some creative ways that can be employed to ensure Ruth has a voice within her family.

To begin this line of discussion, I introduced a set of picture cards to help them both express each of their views regarding how they see their life currently – the here and now. Immediately they both became very engaged in the task together. Ruth was familiar with the use of innovative materials and participated very freely with the use of pictures. John reported he was happy to join in and experiment, but he acknowledged that this was a new approach for him. They were both interested in each other's respective selections (each selected their cards individually) and their narratives about each of their pictures. Through the use of these pictures, we all started to work and communicate together in a way that was a slight surprise to them both, as shown by smiling, laughing and frequent use of eye contact and eye pointing. Ruth selected two pictures and John selected four. We talked through John's pictures first (by mutual consent). He was able to share very honestly why he had chosen each picture and was careful to ensure that Ruth understood completely.

JOHN'S PICTURES AND COMMENTS

1 An aerial view of two people sculling in a boat: 'Team work and yet alone', 'No effective support', 'Need more support from close family'
2 A tractor ploughing a field: 'Up and down', 'Boredom of routine', 'Repetitive nature of activities'
3 Steps leading up and away in a countryside setting: 'Steps to a tunnel', 'Not clear where they are leading – a lot of uncertainty'
4 Multiple multi-coloured transverse brain scans: 'Mental balance', 'Well-being rather than unstable'

RUTH'S SELECTIONS

We looked at Ruth's selections, and together we created some descriptions of each picture that resonated with her. John and I offered possible meanings for each of the cards, and the following are those that were accepted:

1 Two hands holding each other – one adult and one child: 'Supported', 'Rely on others', 'Fed up', 'Not able to look after others – they are looking after me'
2 A woman blowing bubbles underwater: 'Helpless', 'Unable to speak rather than strong'

This equal and visible opportunity provided both Ruth and John with a space to express how they each feel about life now.

Session seven: Ruth and Cathy

After the first session with Ruth and John together, John was going away for a while. Ruth indicated that she would like a session on her own with me. This was an opportunity to genuinely hear from Ruth about how she wanted to start to connect with the world outside her home, building on her developing confidence and helping her to move towards feeling 'strong' despite her physical and communication difficulties.

As Ruth and I had been working together to help her feel that she has choice, control and a voice in the decisions in her life, I was keen to take this further. I wanted to enable her to make the most of her engagement, curiosity and preparedness to open up to new ideas. I reminded Ruth that we are taking small steps, one by one, and that the destination of our work together is not defined simply by the next step we take.

In the spirit of experimentation, I offered Ruth the chance to try a new approach I had learned about. I reflected that this was also an experiment for me which she understood. The approach was Talking Mats (Murphy, Cameron, & Boa, 2013) – a practical and visual way to increase an individual's 'capacity to communicate effectively about things that matter to them'. I saw this as a valid resource to use at this time and could see its potential. Ruth indicated through smiling that she was happy to try this new approach.

I hoped that the Talking Mats session with Ruth would help her to see in a very tangible and visual way how her life is now and how her life could be. There are many Talking Mats topic areas available, and I pre-selected five which I felt might be relevant and a good starting point, given her desire to increase her own self-knowledge and re-connect with life. The choice of these five areas was a way to help Ruth engage with the materials as well as to gain some insights into areas she might be interested in. These were:

1 Self-care
2 Health
3 Leisure (home)
4 Leisure (away) (Figure 3.2)
5 Coping

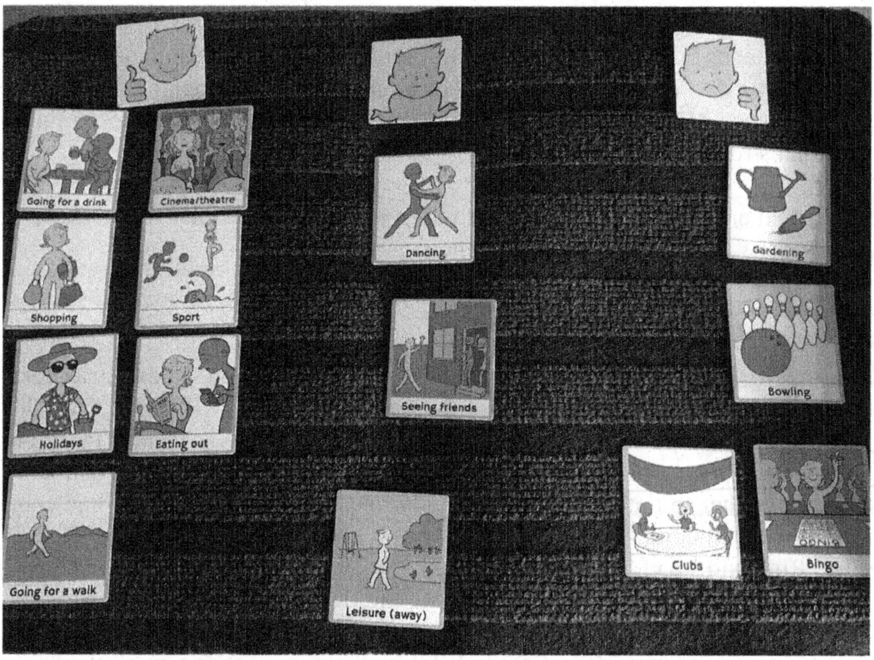

Figure 3.2 Talking Mat: leisure (away)

Source: The symbols are designed and copyrighted to Adam Murphy 2015 and assigned to Talking Mats Ltd. in perpetuity. They may not be reproduced without permission.

I showed Ruth the topics and invited her to choose which one to look at first. For each topic, I (the listener) asked Ruth (the thinker) to place every card I handed her into one of three areas on the mat. I asked her, for example: How do you feel about 'eating out'? Ruth then placed the picture on either the 'Good', 'So-so' or 'Not so good' area.

We moved through the topics in the order listed earlier (Ruth's order choice). Ruth smiled throughout this session whilst handling the cards and placing them where she wanted. For all the topics, I recognised that this was an example of the credulous approach, one in which I was actively attempting to step into her shoes. Ruth made her own decisions, and I could continue to understand *her* world from *her* perspective. I recognised what was important, what was challenging, where she wanted her priorities to be in terms of direction of work, areas she did not want to address and those where she might want to 'dip her toe in'. Through using this technique, together Ruth and I started to highlight via the mats the areas she might like to start to look at in relation to connecting with the outside world.

Session eight: Ruth, John and Cathy

In this session, John joined us again at Ruth's request. The session was open to their concerns and interests. We discussed support structures, cultures and attitudes towards helping within and across their family and friends network (in particular in times of poor health). We referenced the previous joint session at which their perspectives about life now were discussed. Leading on from this, John requested materials that they could use together to be able to discuss their own emotions between themselves outside of our sessions. I agreed to help them access some materials they could use, in particular pictures and photos. A further development was Ruth and John's request to witness other peoples' stories. They had heard of a film called 'My Beautiful Broken Brain' (2014) and wondered whether this was a suitable film to watch. I had seen it but agreed to review it again with them in mind. I also suggested 'The Possibilities are Endless' (2014). I saw a growing curiosity from both Ruth and John not only about the stories and experiences of other people but also about how they themselves might begin to explore possibilities beyond their own situation. I saw my role here as a conduit to opening up their minds to other alternative ways of seeing therapy, help and support. After this session, for external reasons, Ruth and John took a break from our sessions.

MY REFLECTIONS AND LEARNING POINTS

Considering the pathway I have been on with Ruth, there are four key themes relating to PCP, that emerge which I thought would be of interest to share:

1 Highlighting the value of creativity: Experimenting with materials and ideas
2 Negotiating a therapy path: The CPC (decision-making) cycle
3 Providing a voice: Two 'experts' in (and out of) the room
4 Connecting with the world: 'Credulous' listening approach

i) *Highlighting the value of creativity: Experimenting with materials and ideas*

Through PCP counselling, I aim to facilitate clients to conduct experiments that test out their current perceptions, interpretations and constructions of the world. In this way we are both playing the role of 'Person as scientist'. I strive to create an environment in which both the client and I can experiment with approaches and look for options and opportunities outside the therapy room for further experiments beyond our sessions. Because client choice is paramount, I need to ensure that I have access to a wide range of alternative materials, and I am always looking for more. The relationship is a constant joint venture of discovery. Ruth's use of jewellery in our sessions brought a new dimension to our working practice. It was not the pieces of jewellery per se which were so pivotal (although they were key); rather it was the fact that she had selected something from her own world to engage with, and this gave me the confidence that she understood our roles in this therapeutic partnership. The foundations of an equal relationship were being established.

ii) *Negotiating a therapy path: The CPC (decision-making) cycle*

As therapy begins, a relationship develops between two people and a way forward opens up. As a practitioner, I need to pay constant attention to the minutiae of changes that a client makes in response to the work we create together. The CPC cycle is a valuable overarching framework which helps me understand the flow of intervention. The cycle reminds me as a counsellor that options emerge (circumspection), a weighing up of two options becomes evident (pre-emption) and a step in the direction that makes most sense to the client surfaces (control). The client and the counsellor are in the cycle together. Ruth has been at the centre of such a process and thus has helped shape the path of therapy.

iii) *Providing a voice: Two 'experts' in (and out of) the room*

With someone who has severe communication difficulties, I know that the idea of two 'experts' in the room is one in which I need to consistently hold in mind. Through the collaboration with Ruth, I helped her come to recognise that she is the authority in herself and as such has choice and influence. I tried to ensure that Ruth saw herself as having an equal role not just to me as the therapist, but to others in her family and friends network, despite her communication differences. I felt that I was providing the chance for Ruth to embrace this equal if different role within her family through working with her partner and son in different combinations. Making links between the therapy room and the real world provided Ruth with the key to moving forward.

iv) Connecting with the world: 'Credulous' listening approach

Throughout all the sessions with Ruth, I have endeavoured to embrace a 'credulous listening' approach. PCP sees this as the practitioner openly listening to and not making assumptions about the story the client tells and through this lens, making an attempt to step into the shoes of that individual. This type of approach involves the practitioner suspending their own construing as far as possible and subsuming the client's. These skills are at the heart of a PCP approach and are important throughout the therapeutic process. To be able to step into Ruth's shoes, a woman whose communication is severely restricted, I had to pay constant attention to her own personal meaning whilst suspending my own. Through writing this article, I have realised how I have tried to give Ruth options at all stages, whilst also double checking with her that I am not making any unfair assumptions. I have been reminded of the extent to which this is such a feature of how I work with people.

Final thoughts

How does someone make sense of themselves when they have changed so much, including a major shift in their communication abilities? Through working with people like Ruth, I have learned, amongst other things: the value of a creative milieu, the need to help every client find their own voice and means of expression, the importance of providing a forum for experimentation and the significance of credulous listening. I can easily feel daunted when working with people with severe communication difficulties despite my experience and they can of course feel daunted too. But PCP provides a framework which allows me to work through these anxieties. As Brumfitt (2000) says, 'The application of Personal Construct Theory to our understanding of the reactions to stroke and acquired communication problems can offer theoretical insights which make it easier to understand the meaning of the problem to the individual and understand the process the individual experiences in terms of emotional reactions'. She goes on to reflect that 'as an approach to counselling, it (PCP) offers a structure to the recovery process which aids our therapeutic understanding and can only benefit our clients'. The theory acknowledges that we (as counsellor and client) are both in this experience together and that travelling and learning alongside each other is fundamental.

Ruth reports she continues to feel 'stronger', trying out a range of new experiences and connecting more constructively and confidently with her family and friends. The counselling continues at her pace and with her ideas at the core. We may not know what we will eventually achieve, but we know we are moving together in a meaningful direction.

Cathy Sparkes
www.cathysparkes.co.uk

References

Brumfitt, S. (2000). Personal construct theory in stroke and communication problems. In R. Fawcus (Ed.), *Stroke rehabilitation: A collaborative approach*. New Jersey: Wiley-Blackwell.

Collins, E. (2014). *The possibilities are endless*. A Pulse Films Production.
Dalton, P. (1990). Living in the present: The experience of living with amnesia. *Paper presented at the 2nd British conference on PCP*. College of Ripon and York St. John, April 1990.
Dalton, P. (1994). *Counselling people with communication problems*. California: Sage Publications.
Dalton, P., & Dunnett, G. (2005). *A psychology for living: Personal construct theory for professionals and clients* (2nd ed.). New Jersey: Wiley.
Fransella, F. (1972). *Personal change and reconstruction*. London: Academic Press.
Fransella, F., & Dalton, P. (1990). *Personal construct counselling in action*. London: Sage Publications.
Jones, H. (1988). Personal Construct Psychology and counselling: A personal view. In G. Dunnett (Ed.), *Working with people*, Chapter 11. Oxford: Routledge.
Kelly, G. (1955/1991). *The psychology of personal constructs* (Vol. 1 and 2). New York: Norton. Reprinted, London: Routledge.
Murphy, J., Cameron, L., & Boa, S. (2013). *Talking mats: A resource to enhance communication* (2nd ed.). Retrieved from www.talkingmats.com
Parr, S., Byng, S., Gilpin, S., & Ireland, C. (1997). *Talking about aphasia*. Oxford: Open University Press.
Sodderland, L. (2014). *My beautiful broken brain*. Netflix.
Stokes, J. (2009). *Evoke cards*. Retrieved from www.evokecards.com
Sunderland, M., & Engleheart, P. (2015). *Draw on your emotions*. London: Speechmark.
Wilson, P., & Long, I. (2008). *The big book of blobs*. London: Speechmark.

Chapter 4

Supporting families with aphasia to explore relationships

Kate H. Meredith

Introduction

Approximately 320,000 to 350,000 people have an acquired brain injury (ABI) each year in the UK (Headway, 2017). These can be strokes, traumatic brain injuries or other injuries such as tumours and encephalitis. As research increasingly shines light upon the experiences of the family rather than just the individual, we can begin to better understand that there is a relative influence between ABI and families; that is, not only does an ABI affect a family, but that family relationships can also affect the outcome of an ABI. In their extensive literature review of stress and coping in families following brain injury, Verhaeghe, Defloor, and Grypdonck (2005) found that coping ability in family members was positively associated with better recovery in the individual. Norup, Siert, and Lykke Mortensen (2010) also found a correlation between the functional abilities of people with traumatic brain injury in early rehabilitation and the level of self-reported anxiety and depression in relatives.

Families living with aphasia after an ABI face a unique set of challenges. Aphasia can be defined as a disorder of language and communication that can affect a person's ability to understand, speak, read, write and use numbers, but doesn't affect a person's intelligence (Stroke Association, 2019). There are approximately 350,000 people living with aphasia in the UK, over a third of whom are dependent on others for support (Stroke Association, 2019). As rehabilitation professionals, we often turn to families when considering discharge-planning and long-term support for people with aphasia. However, it has been estimated that 30 to 50% of couples divorce within the 5 to 10 years following traumatic brain injuries (Verhaeghe et al., 2005; Wood & Yurdakul, 1997), meaning that those plans and provisions may only be short-to-medium term (although Bowen, Yeates, & Palmer, 2010 warn that these estimates vary and are not dissimilar to divorce rates in the general population). The impact of aphasia on couple relationships specifically has been explored alongside some useful approaches for clinicians to consider (e.g. Lock et al., 2001; Stiell, Naaman, & Lee, 2007; Stiell & Gailey, 2011).

It has been demonstrated that family members of people with ABI experience significantly more psychological distress and are more vulnerable to disruption in family functioning than a normal population (Carnes & Quinn, 2005). In this paper, I argue that there is a benefit to working with families to support them with adjustment to their relationships, with further associated benefits for robust discharge-planning and positive outcomes. In some other health contexts, family therapists may be part of a team and have a role in supporting people to explore their relationships and work towards positive change, but this role is not currently part of a standard neuro-rehabilitation team. The knowledge, skills and experience of an ABI rehabilitation team may be highly developed in many areas but can be relatively reduced when it comes to talking about relationships, which is not always seen as a core part of the work of a rehabilitation team.

Where people experience aphasia after an ABI, the complexity with communication can contribute to increased complexity when exploring relationships and resources, particularly for therapists used to using language as their main tool. Rehabilitation professionals with skills in facilitating communication can therefore be very helpful in this work. Speech and language therapists are usually those with the remit and skills to support people with aphasia in developing their communication.

There is, to date, relatively little literature demonstrating the integration of speech and language therapy and systemic family therapy ideas. Value has been placed on joint work between family therapists and speech and language therapists, or family therapists developing skills working with communication disorders, as existing accounts of such work demonstrate results that are very meaningful for families living with communication disorders following ABI (Bowen et al., 2010; Herrmann, 1989; LarØi, 2003; Nichols, Varchevker, & Pring, 1996; Stiell et al., 2007; Währborg & Borenstein, 1989; Währborg, 1989). Some even question whether a new profession of people with skills in family therapy and neuro-rehabilitation is required (Johnson & McCown, 1997).

I use this article as a space to explore my learning and professional journey as a speech and language therapist and family therapist working with acquired brain injury, neurodisability and communication disorders. I outline some key family therapy concepts and relate these to the field of aphasia, using case examples and contributions from a focus group to demonstrate the use of tools and therapeutic approaches that may be helpful to professionals working systemically with people with aphasia, and for consideration by any rehabilitation professionals. Clearly, I do not have the space here to talk about all of the ideas taught throughout the family therapy training and how these can be relevant to professionals working with aphasia, so I have discussed a select few concepts and therapeutic tools that I think may support many of the people that we work with, in terms of their relationships, adjustment, discharge-planning and quality of life. There is a need for increased exploration of the impact that systemic approaches can have in this area, and so I recommend increased research into the use of these ideas in ABI and aphasia rehabilitation.

Clinical experience

I have worked as a speech and language therapist (SLT) with people with ABI and neurodisability for 13 years. Throughout this time, I have often found myself working with families who are struggling to make sense of their situation and how their lives may look going forward living with brain injury and communication disorders. As an SLT working with people with aphasia, I understood my role as assessing and treating the aphasia at the levels of impairment, activity and participation (World Health Organization, 2001). I involved family members to help me understand the difficulties, use helpful strategies to support the person with aphasia to communicate to their full potential, and develop their own communication skills to enable successful communication. I was strongly influenced by the principles of the social model of aphasia (Byng & Felson Duchan, 2005), believing that factors in the wider environment prevent people with aphasia fully participating in society, and that the involvement of family members helped to share out the responsibility for successful communication. I worked with families to use strategies and tools, from using Total Communication strategies such as gesture and drawing (Pound, Parr, Lindsay, & Woolf, 2000) to developing personalised communication books and using conversation supports such as Talking Mats (www.talkingmats.com). Working with family members therefore became routine for me, but our conversations were mainly in line with the therapeutic agenda that I had set of facilitating positive development in the family's communication skills.

In the specialist neurological rehabilitation centres and community services I have worked in, the families worked with professionals with the knowledge and skills to support people with rehabilitation of their cognition, communication, mobility, continence, independence with activities of daily living and swallowing. But despite the gains that were often made, I wondered if we were at times missing some important opportunities. Compartmentally, skill by skill, people were being rehabilitated. But what I found to be variable (and may be very different in other rehabilitation teams) was the availability of clinicians with the skills, confidence and opportunity to talk to the families about how they had experienced the injury and the acute phase, how their experience was changing, what this meant for them, how this was affecting them, how they saw their future and what was going to promote their resilience as a family to live in a different way. There is a growing body of literature and clinical examples of rehabilitation professionals (neuropsychologists in particular) working with the impact of ABI on self-identity and family identity (e.g. Gracey et al., 2008; Yeates, Gracey, & Collicutt McGrath, 2008; Carroll & Coetzer, 2011; Landau & Hissett, 2008), but I would venture that valuable work and exploration of relationships is not consistent across ABI services. I have worked with therapists, doctors and nurses with highly specialised skills, but even the neuropsychologists have at times found it hard to carve out time for these conversations, given their resource and the cognitive and behavioural assessment and advice that they were also required to provide as part of their role. In teams where no neuropsychologist was available, the absence of these fundamental conversations was even more likely. As discussed earlier, relationships in families can affect long-term outcomes for people with ABI. If we are not enabled, or do not have the capacity, to explore relationships or resources with families following ABI, what opportunities might we be denying our service users?

As I started my training as a family therapist, I began to understand that family therapists were a core part of the multi-disciplinary team in many mental health services, including child and adolescent mental health services, older age psychiatry, eating disorders, couples therapy and addiction services, to name but a few. As I met mental health professionals from these contexts and others, we struggled to understand why in many physical health settings family therapy was not prioritised, despite the significant impact that these illnesses have on the wider system. Stratton (2016) highlights evidence that family therapy is "effective in chronic conditions where it does not make sense to talk of a cure [but] establishing a quality of life through the system of relationships and in a way that recognises and incorporates the condition". My peers and teachers in the family therapy training were intrigued and excited as to what could be brought into the field of ABI and communication disorders.

What is family therapy?

Family therapy (also known as family and systemic psychotherapy) involves a therapist assessing and intervening with a family by asking questions to discuss issues affecting their relationships. The Association for Family Therapy and Systemic Practice (AFT) explains:

> "Family Therapy helps people in close relationship help each other. It enables family members, couples and others who care about each other to express and explore thoughts and emotions safely, to understand each other's experiences and views, appreciate each other's needs, build on strengths and make useful changes in their relationships and their lives. Individuals also can find Family Therapy helpful, as an opportunity to reflect and strengthen important relationships."
>
> (www.aft.org.uk)

Family therapists draw upon a wide range of theoretical models when working with families. I now discuss some of the concepts and tools that I feel are useful to consider when working with people with aphasia and their families. I learned about these concepts through my family therapy training, but it should be noted that family therapy is a broad theoretical church that has been influenced by, and influences, other models, and some of these ideas are well understood within other models, sometimes using different names and terms. Many of the interventions I discuss in this article are based on the psychotherapeutic default of spoken language, but can be adapted in many ways for people with receptive language difficulties, particularly if the clinician is used to using Total Communication approaches (Pound et al., 2000) and adapting communication to the needs of the person with aphasia.

The family life cycle

The family life cycle is a model for thinking about family development (Carter & McGoldrick, 1988). Families develop through key stages, such as leaving home, becoming a couple, starting a family, becoming a family with adolescents, launching children and moving into later family life (including retirement, illness and death). Moving among stages involves transition, which can be challenging and requires family adjustment. Perhaps we can all think of times in our own families where moving through the cycle has been positive and a cause for celebration, and also times when transition has been difficult, complicated or distressing. Getting 'stuck' in a life cycle stage can stop us from developing appropriately, or cause further distress or illness.

The family life cycle can be disrupted by 'stressors'. 'Vertical' stressors are passed down through the generations of the family and can include family secrets, rules and taboos. 'Horizontal' stressors come from outside the family and can include events and processes such as illness, divorce and bankruptcy. Families can experience stress and anxiety when either type of stressor is present, which may affect emotional transactions and the emergence of individual symptoms.

Aphasia can be conceptualised as a horizontal stressor that the family is required to adapt to and move on with, in order to fulfil further life cycle goals. If the family becomes 'stuck', it is harder to grow and complete the development tasks necessary to move on to a following stage (Leaf, 1993). By asking about both the immediate and wider family life cycle, and considering the stages and transitions that are in process or imminent, we can assess the impact of aphasia on the family. We can help the family to think about ways to fulfil stages of the cycle, prepare for transition or complete transition to the next phase of the cycle by countering its influence. By not considering the family processes that were taking place before the onset of the aphasia, we risk viewing families as homogenous, without considering their resources and constraints in managing the aphasia and its influences. A useful way to begin to explore the family life cycle is discussed next.

Genograms and ecomaps

Genograms (McGoldrick & Gerson, 1985) and ecomaps (Hartman, 1995) are tools for visually representing a family structure and other systems relevant to the family. Many health professionals are familiar with representing information pictorially or symbolically for a person with aphasia and know that the permanence of writing and drawing supports comprehension and retention. The use of a genogram or ecomap provides a visual tool to use with people who may benefit from a visual or multi-modal approach. Additionally, photographs could be used

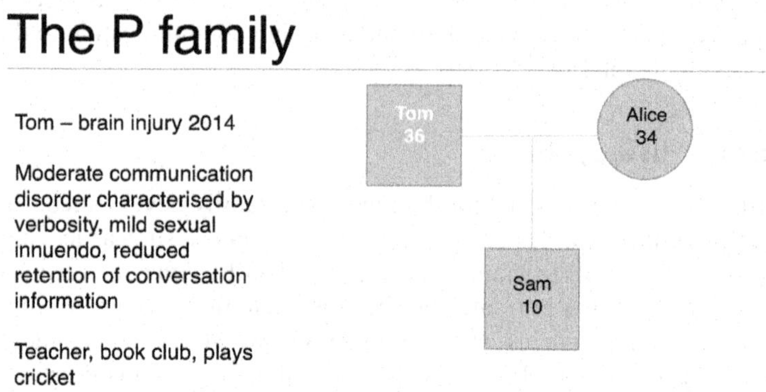

Figure 4.1 Example of a two-generation family genogram

here rather than, or in addition to, written names, to further support comprehension difficulties.

Family therapists often try to include at least three generations in the genogram, to better understand the family structure, relationships and patterns that may emerge. For many professionals, finding out information about the immediate family may be important, but the genogram might not extend beyond this, giving us the two-generation information illustrated in Figure 4.1.

We can certainly work with this information and look at the needs of the immediate, 'nuclear' (Minuchin, 1974) family. We might think about inviting Alice in for communication therapy sessions, to participate in therapy and extend strategies into conversation among the three of them in evenings and at weekends. We might ask Sam to come in after school for the same reasons. We might look at setting communication goals not just around basic needs such as toileting on the ward, asking for food and drink and indicating pain, but also around teaching, reading and cricket. But if we spent a little more time, completing a three-generation genogram (Figure 4.2), and asking about the relationships in the family, and issues including closeness, distance and health, what else might we discover?

The information we now have shows us a clearer representation of this family's stage of the life cycle and the transitions that they are currently experiencing that may be further complicated by Tom's injury and the communication disorder. We can be more aware of many aspects of family life that can be important for us to understand and useful for us to work with, for example:

- The recent family losses (indicated by crosses next to Mike and Sue signifying death, and the slanted lines between Kay and Will's marriage, signifying divorce), and reduced family support for Alice
- The feelings Sam has about visiting his father in hospital, and whether there is a better context to meet in, if information is needed in a child-friendly

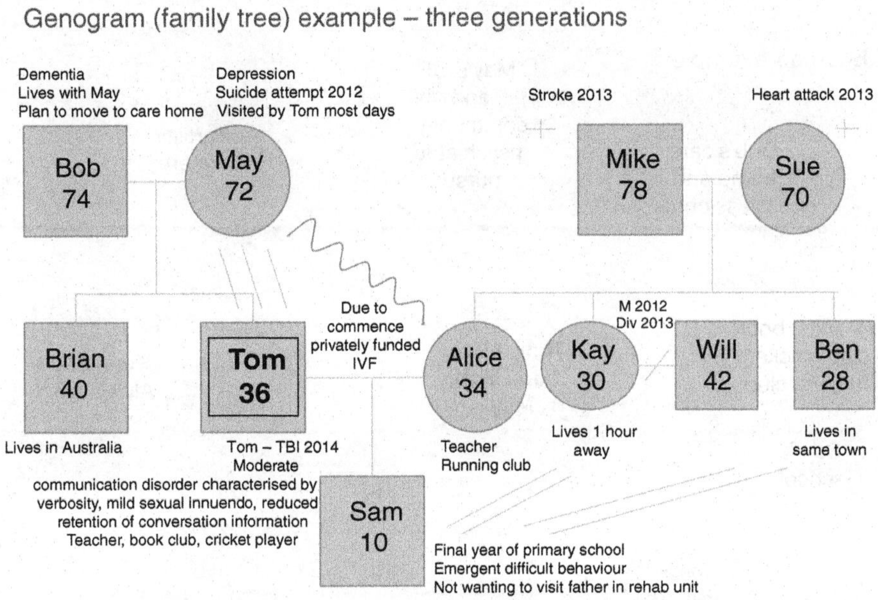

Figure 4.2 Example of a three-generation family genogram

format, or if sessions to enable Sam to ask questions and say what is on his mind would be welcomed by the family

- The strong relationships that Sam has with his aunt and uncle (indicated by multiple straight lines), and how these people might be important supports for him
- The difficult relationship that Alice has with Tom's mother, May (indicated by squiggly line), and the complex support needs that May and Bob have, that Tom has previously fulfilled
- The ways in which we might be able to work with Tom to continue communication with May and Bob despite the difficulty visiting in person whilst on the ward

These pertinent details may emerge from conversations with any member of the rehabilitation team during assessments, and it is essential that teams find ways within their services of sharing this information sensitively, for the benefit of the family. There may also be standardised assessments that make space for these questions to be asked but may not be routinely covered during the assessment process, for fear of causing offence or bringing up sensitive material that team members may not feel comfortable discussing in more depth.

By asking permission to ask what might be difficult questions, we can raise sensitive subjects and vastly increase our understanding of the family life cycle. The question "Have you had any more children or pregnancies?" enables us to

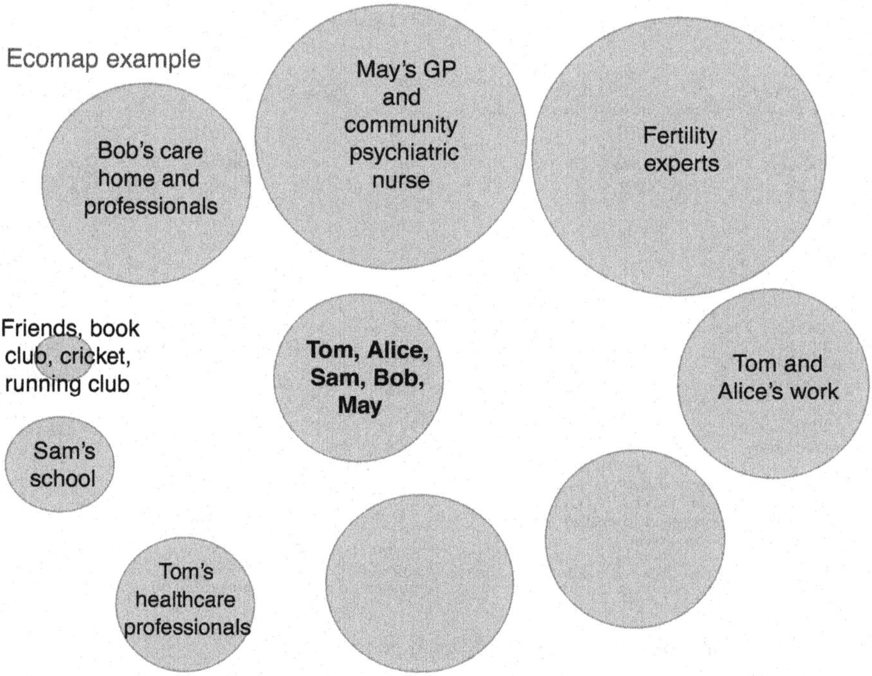

Figure 4.3 Family ecomap example

hear from Alice that Tom and Alice have tried for many years to have a second child and were shortly to commence IVF treatment. This enables us to support Alice to ask questions of Tom's medical team regarding his prognosis and capacity to consent to the IVF process that she is strongly committed to.

If we go further and complete an ecomap (Hartman, 1995) (Figure 4.3), we can look at the systems that the family is currently involved with.

Tom and his immediate family are placed in the middle, and we have learned about the services they are required to interact with over the course of a week. A circle has been drawn for each group, based on the intensity of the interactions and the demands placed on Tom and Alice. We can ask whether the space these services take up is positive or negative; which circles they would like to be bigger, smaller or even absent. We can even draw two or three empty circles and ask, "If these were to be filled with people or services providing extra support that you would value, who would be in them?" Again, photographs or drawings could be used here to further support receptive difficulties. In services with neuropsychology readily available, these issues may be addressed as part of their assessment, but any health professional could complete this exercise with the family. This exercise enables greater understanding on the part of the healthcare professionals and the family of who else to involve, what the family priorities are, what the functional goals for communication therapy might be, and where there is potential for isolation. For example, we might find:

- The communication with these systems was previously shared between Tom and Alice; now Alice is largely responsible for communicating with everyone. We can see why our offers of evening therapy sessions or mid-week family meetings might not be received as enthusiastically as we thought they might be, and why our suggestions of functional communication goals around communicating with cricket friends might not feel the biggest priority.
- Both Tom and Alice are conscious of the need for greater communication with the school at present, given the difficulties with Sam's behaviour that are emerging and his pending transition from primary school to secondary school. However, given the other demands on Alice's time, this is complicated to achieve. Are there other members of the family who could support Tom and Alice to communicate with the school about Sam's needs, or to support them with their other commitments to free up space for them to communicate with the school?
- Alice feels the need to step in for Tom with communication with May's GP, community psychiatric nurse, Bob's care home and health professionals. However, we might be able to support Alice and Tom to think about who else might be able to be involved, and whether Tom's brother Brian might be able to communicate with these systems via email, to support his parents' needs and allow Tom and Alice to focus on other areas.
- Tom's friends from work and his social activities might be very keen to visit and be involved in Tom's therapy where appropriate; however, they have had difficulty making contact with Alice as she hasn't been able to return their calls because of the other priorities. We might be able to support Tom to make contact with them himself and invite them in to see him, to reduce the isolation he might otherwise experience.

Social constructionism and narrative therapy

The concept of social construction (e.g. Anderson & Goolishian, 1988; Tomm, 1998; Burr, 2003) has had a significant impact on my understanding of the impact of aphasia and other communication disorders. Its premise is that our knowledge of the world is constructed socially. That is, it is constructed through language in social communities. The interactions that we have with other people influence the beliefs that we hold and the language that we use in spoken and written conversations. As we have these conversations, we construct truth rather than discover it. We tell stories that make sense to us and the beliefs that we hold and, if these beliefs and the version of the truth that we tell fits for others, then the stories get re-told. As communities, we retain useful constructions of events, objects and relationships, and those that are not useful, we discard (Burr, 2003).

Social constructionism has influenced a range of therapies, including narrative therapy (White & Epston, 1990), where the idea is continued that people make sense of their world by telling, and listening to, stories about their lives. These stories are enormously powerful: conversations can shape new realities, and weak voices have little power to change stories told. These weaker, untold stories are known as 'subjugated narratives'.

We may all be able to think of a story that has been told about us that didn't fit our experience when we heard it, and that we found difficult to challenge. Our parents may have told stories about us being terrible teenagers, our partners may have shared stories with our friends about our atrocious driving, or our children may have told their friends or grandparents how mean and unfair we are to them. Much of the time we might be able to engage in the story-telling to present a different view, perhaps by explaining that we thought rationing sweets before bedtime was good parenting rather than a campaign to induce misery in our children. In other situations, it becomes more difficult to challenge the story being told. The examples that the storyteller has to hand begin to add up, and the examples we bring to the table where we were rational teenagers or careful drivers drop away and a narrative is constructed where we are defined in a way that we don't feel represents the truth.

As I learned about these concepts, their significance to people with aphasia was immediately evident to me. Not only did people with aphasia have such reduced opportunity to tell stories and challenge versions of the truth that did not fit for them, but also, in my experience, they were less likely to be believed or taken seriously when they were successful. When a person's communication is affected by changes to their language, speech or a cognitive impact on the way that they communicate, it is not uncommon for assumptions to be made about changes in intelligence and personality. Readers may have observed conversation partners speaking to people with aphasia as they might to a child, an elderly person or a person with a hearing impairment, even when they have many years of experience working in a setting with such clients. Indeed, this has been a common complaint to me from people with aphasia during my clinical work. The explicit message is given out to trainees and family members that aphasia does not affect intelligence, but the implicit messages associated with a clinician's tone of voice, impatience or failure to use the conversation supports that will empower a person with aphasia to participate in a conversation tell a different story. A focus group I facilitated with partners of people with communication disorders for my Family Therapy MSc dissertation (Meredith, 2012) allowed me to capture the following quote, from a woman whose husband had a relatively mild communication disorder:

> P2: I do miss this kind of easy kind of conversation . . . sometimes I find I don't take him as seriously as I would have done before. . . . Like, if he says something and I doubt it, and he's sometimes right, what he's saying, and I go "Really? Are you sure?" whereas I never would have doubted something that he'd have said before . . . you just don't seem to give them as much credit. . . . I just sort of think "Are you sure about that?" whereas I wouldn't have doubted it before.
>
> (Meredith, 2012, p. 28)

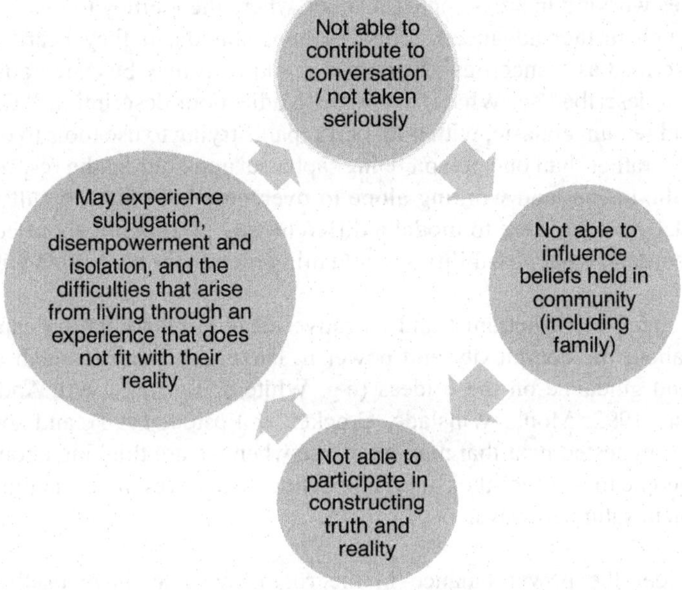

Figure 4.4 Potential implications of not showing respect to people with aphasia in their attempts to communicate

This woman was so generous in her honesty with me and the rest of the group, and I felt it captured perfectly my impression that, even when able to overcome the obstacle of aphasia and communicate a message, people with aphasia may not be given the respect and confidence of conversation partners that they once were. The implications of this may be as depicted in Figure 4.4.

When considering language as a tool of social power, we must also consider the labels and shorthand that we use, for reasons of habit or ease. As health professionals, we find ourselves talking about people in a variety of settings, using different terminology. In some settings, 'patient' seems an appropriate term; in another 'client' is preferable. Some of us may ask people we are working with about their preferences for such terminology; others may not have considered this much of an issue. As we have seen from the above, the language we use can be of great significance if it places people into a story or reality that does not fit for them. If we ascribe a role to people – be that victim, patient, client or survivor – do we situate people in relation to their ABI forever more? Furthermore, if the shorthand we use is even more defining of the person (e.g. "he's aphasic"; "she's brain-injured"), is there room for anything else? In certain areas of the health services, we have perhaps been a little slower to catch on to this. Colleagues working in some mental health settings have started this journey a little earlier, and the contexts in which they work can be more sensitive to these labels (although similarly to physical health settings, practice can be variable). Colleagues working in areas such as cancer, where the journey to externalisation is also much further advanced, might perhaps shudder if they heard a person being described as 'cancerous'. Body tissue and cells may be cancerous; people are seldom described so. What if we were to adjust our descriptions? Conversations could remain aphasic, with both participants trying to use tools to overcome the aphasia rather than one person being 'aphasic' and holding the responsibility, possibly the blame, and working alone to overcome both the difficulty and the defining label. If we were to model a different way of thinking about communication disorders, what possibilities would this generate for the people with whom we work?

Using social constructionist and narrative ideas in rehabilitation can help us to think about the complexity and power in language. There is much excellent writing and guidance on these ideas (e.g. White & Epston, 1990; Anderson & Goolishian, 1992; Monk, Winslade, Crocket, & Epston, 1996), and some brief points are suggested next that may be of use when we are thinking about how to support people to reauthor their lives and define themselves in non-pathologising, non-problem saturated ways.

1 Consider the power balance in the room. We may have useful clinical expertise, but our clients are experts in their own situation, their own story (Anderson & Goolishian, 1992). What steps can we take to address the often-disempowering context that we work in?
2 Hear the problem fully; understand how it makes people feel. This may involve booking out extra time, the use of supported conversation techniques, involving a third party (e.g. an SLT) who can focus on facilitating communication, or skilling yourself up to a level where you feel you can confidently and flexibly use a variety of tools to support a person with aphasia to get their version of events across.
3 Externalise the problem; that is, work to separate the problem from the person (White & Epston, 1990). The person and the injury are not the same thing, but our language does not always support this distinction. Can we move from "(s)he's aphasic" to "the aphasia"? Or to characterise it even further, using capitals and dropping the definite article? Consider the difference between "John's become really lazy" vs. "The brain injury steals John's energy", or "Don't tell Sarah; she won't remember" vs. "Sarah has to fight Forgetfulness with a notebook and diary". As we further externalise the problem, is there perhaps another name that the person would use for 'Aphasia' that better fits with their reality?
4 Understand the influence of the problem on the person, the couple, the family (White & Epston, 1990). When is Aphasia most or least powerful, silencing, or disruptive to family life? What does it try to do to people, to relationships? Are there times in their day/week when Aphasia seems overwhelmingly present, or when it has less of an impact? When the problem is less problematic, or when they find it easier to manage?

5 Explore the influence that the family can have on Aphasia (White & Epston, 1990). What happens to Aphasia when Tess draws a picture for her father? When Rachel checks that she has interpreted her husband correctly before moving on? Or when Daniel gives his mother more time in conversation? Is it more or less present in the room; is it more or less powerful? When have they managed to outsmart Aphasia? When they were more in control of Aphasia? When they were able to ask for help in outwitting Aphasia? When they were able to put Aphasia away for the evening? Who/what helped? How did they know they had 'got one over' on this intruder in their relationship?

6 Have there been other times that the family had to unite against something difficult (White & Epston, 1990)? How did they do this? What are the tools that they used then, and how might these be used now to fight the influence of Aphasia in their family?

7 Reflect on times in the recent past where communication has been easier, by looking for unique outcomes (White & Epston, 1990). What was different about these times? What were people doing that was so successful? Can it be named, shared, drawn upon? Where else can we see this happening? How could we all work against Aphasia to see more examples of this in the present and future? How could we see improved communication more often in this context, or moving to other contexts, or different relationships?

8 Can we add permanence to this new narrative of successful communication? Therapeutic letters (White & Epston, 1990) can help us to give weight to conversations we have had in therapy. We can witness subjugated stories (White & Epston, 1990), give permanence to alternative narratives, and historicise progress by capturing in ink the conversations we have had and the emerging person and relationships we can see when Aphasia becomes less of an identifier.

There are already some good examples of externalisation in healthcare. The well-known 'Race For Life' campaign in 2013 showed a group of people using the phrase, "Cancer, we're coming to get you", as well as hurling insults at the disease. The illness was seen not as integral to a person but external, an enemy for a community to rise up and fight against. In an eating disorders context, the 'Anti-Anorexia league' has brought together "communities of people who have taken a stand against the oppressive regimes of anorexia and bulimia in their own lives and are prepared to share their stories with others who are struggling with these problems" (Epston & Madigan, 1995).

What ideas from these campaigns could we be influenced by and use in the fields of ABI and communication disorders, that externalise the injuries and disorders as something affecting society rather than being integral to a person's identity?

Resilience

I include resilience here as I learned about it through my family therapy training, but therapists from a wide range of schools explore resilience, including but not limited to cognitive behavioural therapy (Padesky & Mooney, 2012), and 'resilient therapy' itself (Hart, Blincow, & Thomas, 2007). There is the understanding that resilience may be "strongly influenced by people's patterns of interpersonal relationships [and therefore] relevant to the field of family therapy" (Rutter, 1999). In their critical review of the impact of brain injury on the family, Perlesz, Kinsella, and Crowe (1999) found that research attends more to relatives' stress and burden than exploring resilience and positive family outcomes. There is more recent literature on family coping after ABI (e.g. Verhaeghe et al., 2005; Carnes & Quinn, 2005), but I note this study in particular for the attention Perlesz and colleagues (1999) bring to researchers' tendencies to neglect resilience factors. This fits with the complexity I have encountered in clinical work. Despite my appreciation of the nature of family therapy being to "help people mobilise the strengths of their relationships so as to make disturbing symptoms unnecessary or less problematic" (Stratton, 2016), I have at times been organised by the need to highlight the unique difficulties experienced by families with aphasia, and needed to bring my attention back to the family's ability to manage such a disruptive intrusion to family life by exploring factors supporting their resilience. Resilience can be described as "the process of, capacity for, or outcome of successful adaptation despite challenging circumstances" (Masten, Best, & Garmezy, 1990). Unfortunately for families living with aphasia, factors that support resilience with illness and injury are often based in communication. Revenson (2003) found that partner coping during chronic illness is influenced by many factors, including the ability to communicate reciprocally with the ill partner. Rolland (1994) believed that couples who can communicate openly, directly and sensitively can better cope with chronic disorders, whilst reciprocal communication and affective relations have been found to be important factors in family coping (Anderson, Parmenter, & Mok, 2002; Florian, Katz, & Lahav, 1989; Kreutzer, Gervasio, & Camplair, 1994).

We can understand that open, reciprocal communication is associated with coping during illness, but this is not always possible. How do couples and families living with communication difficulties manage issues such as establishing boundaries around the illness and achieving balance in their relationships? By asking questions about resilience, we can think with people about the protective factors they may have internally (in their character), or externally (in their environment), that support their resilience at this time.

A range of coping mechanisms have been found to be utilised by family members following ABI, although some of the research related to these findings was conducted some time ago and should be interpreted with caution. Emotion-oriented coping mechanisms include denial, avoidance through the use of alcohol or medications and faith (Panting & Merry, 1970; Romano, 1974; Mauss-Clum & Ryan, 1981, cited in Verhaeghe et al., 2005; Livingston, 1987; Minnes, Graffi, Nolte, Carlson, & Harrick, 2000). Problem-oriented coping mechanisms include giving up work (Hall et al., 1994), yet this can also increase social isolation and reduce financial resources. Problem-solving coping mechanisms include seeking social support and taking on the roles previously held by the person with the brain injury (Hallett, Zasler, Maurer, & Cash, 1994; Minnes et al., 2000); however, partners of people with severe communication disorders have been found in the past to isolate themselves from social networks to avoid placing their partner or friends in an embarrassing situation (Kinsella & Duffy, 1978, cited in Michallet, Tétreault, & Le Dorze, 2003). Divorce can be seen as either an emotion-oriented coping mechanism or a problem-oriented coping mechanism (Verhaeghe et al., 2005).

To explore family resilience, using ideas from the aforementioned research, we might ask some of the following questions:

- Many families might feel unable to cope in this situation; others might find ways to manage despite the difficulties faced. How would you describe your experience?
- What strategies do you have that are working to help you manage at this time? Can you name any?
- Would other people say you have strategies? How would they describe them?
- What protective factors do you have, to support your resilience at this time?
- (If they feel that they are coping) What is it about your character that is helping you to cope? If this is difficult, think of what your best friend might say about your character and why it is that you can manage this situation in the way you are?
- What is present within your environment that supports you in this situation? (e.g. specific friends, hobbies, employment, pets, etc.)
- (If they feel that they are coping). What has surprised you about the ways in which you have coped so far?

Reference to a genogram can also be helpful when exploring resilience. We may see that families have been through very difficult times before, that we can gently enquire about. My focus group (Meredith, 2012) gave me examples of times when the couples had been through complexity and tragedy and had found a way through it:

> P4: Where she's been ill for so long, I think, in a sort of roundabout way, that's sort of helped me in way, ... I'm so used to her being ill, so this is just like another stepping stone. . . . And losing our son, it's just sort of been constant bad luck, so, coping with all those things, this is just sort of another thing that's happened, . . . and I just sort of take it day by day, and you learn things every day. . . .
>
> P2: We lost our first child; he was stillborn, and that definitely makes you stronger, I think, as a couple, because you share that and nobody else shares that, it's a, yeah, so a few things, I think, yeah, those things do help to make you stronger and get through things, I think.
>
> (Meredith, 2012, pp. 40–41)

The partners spoke of strategies learned and strong foundations in their relationships formed through shared experiences, that may be helpful to them as they navigate this situation.

As with so many conversations we have, this would need to be sensitively handled. Staff need not only the opportunity, training and skills, but also the space for exploring the issues that arise in supervision and reflection. Asking about coping can imply that people *should* cope, or that saying that they are not coping is to fail. We might see people managing relatively well and feel that they are coping, whereas they might feel that they are simply surviving. But to not ask about resilience may also be letting them down. By drawing attention to these issues, people can receive positive feedback regarding their ability to survive such a complex event as living with aphasia in the family, and build on the skills and strategies that they are using. They can reflect on what they have learned from previous experience that they can use now. They can also feel supported to place value on the activities and relationships that can be conceptualised as internal and external protective factors, whether they be walking the dog, meditation, speaking with friends or enjoying a comedy programme.

Combining skills from SLT and family therapy

I mentioned at the beginning of this piece the evidence that family therapists with experience working with communication disorders such as aphasia, or joint work between family therapists and SLTs can produce results that are very meaningful for families living with communication disorders following ABI (Bowen et al., 2010; Herrmann, 1989; LarØi, 2003; Nichols et al., 1996; Stiell et al., 2007; Währborg & Borenstein, 1989; Währborg, 1989). However, in 13 years working in ABI, I have only ever personally encountered this joint work once, with a neuropsychologist who had also trained as a family therapist and provided input to the community rehabilitation service I worked in at the time. Working with him as an SLT was the inspiration for my training in family therapy, as I supported the communication of the person with aphasia in communicating with his wife about his fears for their relationship following his stroke. Since I have trained in this area, I have now learned of two other SLTs working in ABI who are keen to complete the training, which is very encouraging (and there may, of course, be many more). I feel that this is a training that fits so well with the role of SLT that I would encourage any SLT to consider it, as SLTs are so often given insights into the relationships of the people with whom we work that some other health professionals might not be, because of the nature of our work and the relatively private context in which it often takes place (in contrast to a gym, bedside or shower room, for example). What we then do with those opportunities depends not only on the time available to us, but also the knowledge, skills and confidence we have to address sensitive and complex issues regarding relationships.

Over the years, I have supported many people with aphasia to develop or implement communication strategies to communicate with family members or professionals about their concerns. Relationally, these have varied widely and have included communicating fears of relationship breakdown, supporting partners and health professionals to communicate about erectile dysfunction, and supporting people with aphasia to ask children about things that mattered to both of them. I remember these families (and so many others) very clearly for the sense of privilege I felt, to be involved with a family discussing such personal issues. However, had I had my family therapy training by this stage, what might the opportunities have been? I now look back at the case of Barry and Kay (names changed), giving a short summary of the work completed and some ideas that I would now be able to use if I had been able to implement my dual training with them.

Barry and Kay

Barry and Kay had been partners for approximately 12 years but had never lived together or been interested in being married. Barry had a stroke that resulted in severe expressive aphasia and moderate receptive aphasia, with a degree of cognitive-communication disorder and apraxia of speech. Kay visited the ward daily and was a keen and strong advocate for Barry's needs. The discharge plan was for Barry to live with Kay and was briefly confirmed by the key worker and occupational therapist (OT) on admission to the unit and again in the family meeting, and all plans were made with this discharge destination in mind. As a rehabilitation team, we felt very confident of Kay's ability to support Barry on discharge and were not particularly concerned when he opted to have Kay support him with his showering each day rather than participate in personal care rehabilitation with the OTs and nurses. We had felt that with intensive rehabilitation, Barry could become independent with this skill, but he declined, and Kay reported that he had always been very private and would not have wanted to shower with strangers, and after all, she would support him with showering on discharge. Weekend leave was successfully trialled at Kay's home, with her supporting Barry with these tasks.

Barry seemed worried at times and, through the use of supported conversation techniques (Kagan, 1998; Lock et al., 2001), I learned that he was concerned about his relationship with Kay. I gained his permission to raise this with Kay, who dismissed the concerns immediately when I spoke with her separately. I fed this back to Barry and could see that he was not completely reassured. I enquired further about the nature of his concerns, and he was able to communicate that he was scared she would leave him. Again, with permission, I raised this with Kay, and she said that this was not going to happen and told me how much she loved him. I fed this back to Barry, and he communicated that he wished to proceed with the discharge plan. The team was made aware of this but we all felt reassured and discharge-planning continued. Barry was referred to community therapy for SLT only, as Kay told us that she would take care of all of Barry's personal cares, meal preparation and shopping.

On the last day of Barry's admission to the unit, Kay brought in gifts for the rehabilitation team, and she and Barry left together as planned. In the two days that followed, Kay did not respond to telephone messages left to check how things were going at home. We then received a telephone call from the social worker explaining that Kay had called her to inform her that Barry needed to be rehoused as she could not support him with his care needs and wanted to end the relationship. We were not able to make contact with Kay and received little information, but understood from the community SLT that Barry was then placed in a residential care setting, because of his needs for support with all personal care, meal preparation and shopping. As a team, we were deeply saddened by this news. The privacy that Barry had sought from the rehabilitation team and our confidence that Kay was able to complete this role meant that he was now likely to need his care needs supported by carers for the longer term, without the option of further intensive rehabilitation, and was living in a setting that was the last place he had wanted to be.

As I trained in family therapy, this case came back to mind frequently. How might I have addressed this had I had the knowledge and skills I gained during my family therapy training? What would the impact have been? I will, of course, never know. However, I can reflect on the importance of opening communication channels between people rather than acting as a go-between. I can consider how some additional preparations for a conversation between the two of them, possibly with another SLT or psychologist supporting Barry's communication, could have opened up possibilities for exploring the nature of Barry's doubts and the need Kay felt to be so unwavering in her support. I would have needed to seek permission to have a conversation about the relationship with both of them but then might have been able to explore this in more detail. For example:

"Kay, Barry has shown us that he has some concerns, some fears, about your relationship ending after he leaves hospital. Could you tell me what you think is behind Barry's fears?" (*N.B. I could also have worked with Kay to present written, spoken and drawn options to Barry of the ways he might be worried, if this was a more appropriate route to go down, as opposed to the circular question (Cecchin, 1987) used here, where the aim is to ask Kay to think about how Barry might be feeling rather than for Barry to communicate those feelings directly. Both routes could be helpful.*)

[Listening to Kay's responses, writing down key words and using drawing to support Barry's comprehension. Recapping to reflect Kay's expressed ideas and also to support Barry's comprehension. Using supported conversation techniques of shorter sentences, pauses, written support, drawing, gesture and facial expression.]

"Barry, Kay *[point to Kay]* has told you *[gesture of speech]* that she loves you *[gesture of love, written word, drawing of heart]*. Kay says she will support you in her home *[draw Kay's home with Barry and Kay inside]* when you leave hospital *[draw arrow from hospital to Kay's home]*. However, I wonder *[facial expression and gesture indicating me wondering]* if I can see that you *[gesture]* are still worried *[facial expression and written word]*? How worried are you, on a scale of 0 to 10 *[draw visual analogue scale, using pictures of happy and worried faces]*, with 10 being most worried *[point to worried face and 10]* and 0 being not worried at all *[point to happy face and 0]*?"

"Kay, Barry has shown us that he is still 8/10 worried. Could we spend some time thinking about this? Some partners of people on the ward have told me that they find the shift in relationship after stroke complicated; that it is difficult going from being someone's partner and lover to also being their carer. Is this something that has occurred to you? How is being a carer similar or different to the relationship you and Barry had before the stroke?"

[Listening to Kay's responses, writing down key words and using drawing to support Barry's comprehension. Recapping to reflect Kay's expressed ideas and also to support Barry's comprehension. Using supported conversation techniques of shorter sentences, pauses, written support, drawing, gesture and facial expression.]

"Kay, you have told us that you and Barry had a lot of fun as a couple; that life was lived out and about and mainly at the pub with friends, each returning to your own home most nights and once or twice a week to each other's homes. We know that you have offered to support Barry with living with you, helping him to get up in the mornings and get washed and dressed, cooking his meals and doing his shopping and laundry. Barry has told us that since he no longer drinks alcohol and finds group conversation and noisy environments challenging, he does not wish to spend his days at the pub. Do you have any thoughts about how this might impact on your relationship and the life you chose to lead prior to the stroke, or your identity as a couple? If your best friend were here, what might she say the impact would be?"

And so on the conversation might have gone. As Barry's SLT, I knew all the foregoing information about their relationship, but the way I felt able to talk about the relationship with them was very constrained compared with how I might feel able to approach the subject now. I can't know how the conversation would have gone, and whether the outcome for Barry and Kay would have been different, but I can hypothesise that with the space to discuss these issues as a couple, they may have felt more able to talk about some of the fears or ambivalence that they had for their life ahead, and may even have been able to discuss other living arrangements that enabled Barry to have the support he needed but with less pressure on Kay to be the sole provider of this support.

It is not uncommon in my practice for ideas to be shared about the strength of the couple relationship and the ability to survive this complex period. These often come from the musings of health professionals, but in my focus group (Meredith, 2012) more examples were shared by the partners of the people with communication disorders:

P1: When the fog started to clear a bit, he went through a spell where he thought I was leaving him. . . . He wasn't sleeping, and in the end I said to him, "Look, are you worried about something?" and he said, "Well, you should know . . . you're leaving me" and I don't know where it had come from. P2: But it's a natural thing to think, though.

P3: I think at the back of their brain they are thinking probably because they are ill, you might leave them [P2 and P1 agree] – 'Cos sometimes I look into [his] eyes and I see there, "Are you going to leave me now?" . . . That's how it feels; I say, "I'm here, I'm coming back tomorrow" . . . reassuring that I'll be around.

P2: He has actually said to me, "You can go and find someone else; you don't have to stay with me", and I've had to say, "Don't be so silly", and he laughs and says, "That's what they say on the telly; I thought I'd better say it", but I don't know if he might have meant it [group agrees] and is covering it up with that.

(Meredith, 2012, p. 31)

For many of us, our family relationships are some of the very most important issues in our lives. To have aphasia following an ABI, to have anxieties about the ability of our spousal relationships to survive and *not* to be given the opportunity to discuss them may be more distressing than the conversations that would follow with the time and space to think these ideas through.

Working with children

I have largely focused on the couple relationship in this paper, for the reasons that I am unable to cover all family dynamics and because partners experience increased distress, depression, anxiety, poorer health and less stable relationships compared with other family members (Blais & Boisvert, 2007; Bowen, 2007; Kreutzer et al., 1994; Norup et al., 2010; Perlesz, Kinsella, & Crowe, 2000). I do not have the space here to fully explore the issues faced when working with parents who have aphasia, but I wish to make a few brief points. Healthcare professionals often have well-developed skills for engaging children in therapy sessions, and children of any age can benefit from being able to ask healthcare professionals questions about their parents' difficulties and sharing their concerns. They can find some of the tools discussed so far (e.g. genograms and ecomaps) interesting, particularly when they are asked to be useful to the session by providing information about their family or using their drawing skills. It is common in family therapy for children to remain fairly quiet in initial sessions, but my experience is that they are almost always listening and will be unable to resist the urge to join in at times. They are therefore likely to be influenced by the way that we are talking about aphasia. We can take these opportunities to be curious about their position and what it means for them at their stage of the life cycle – we are talking about a very wide age range here, and the impact will be very different for a toddler than for a child shortly to leave the family home to go to university, for example. We can take the opportunity to attend to our language and the positive connotations we can make. We need to be sensitive to children taking parental roles (Byng-Hall, 2008) and becoming a part of the parental subsystem (Minuchin, 1974), the implications for the roles that they are required to complete and the support they are required to give. We need to note and increase opportunities that can arise in sessions to protect the child's role and strengthen the parental subsystem, particularly in cases where linguistic and/or cognitive challenges can potentially disempower parents. We can be active in considering which sessions are appropriate for children to be a part of, and where there might be advantages to holding parent-only sessions to discuss sensitive topics that children do not need to witness. In services where there is not a clinician able to meet with a child to discuss their parent's communication difficulties, ecomaps can be an enormously useful tool in considering the need for signposting children to school services or other services that can help.

Conclusion

Aphasia carries a unique set of complications that health professionals can anticipate and address to support people and families. I have given some ideas in this chapter regarding the implementation of specific therapy ideas for the work of rehabilitation teams with families with aphasia, but what can services and individual health professionals do more broadly, to continue to develop skills working with families?

This volume of *Psychotherapy and Aphasia: Interventions for Emotional Well-being and Relationships* will, I'm sure, give us examples of a variety of psychotherapeutic approaches being useful to families living with aphasia, and I am delighted to think that there is ongoing, increasing recognition of the need for approaches to look at supporting people with aphasia to work psychotherapeutically. As I indicated at the beginning of this article, questions have previously been raised as to whether more professionals working in neuro-rehabilitation services should complete the four-year, masters-level training in family therapy (Bowen, 2007), or if a new profession of people with skills in family therapy and neuro-rehabilitation is required (Johnson & McCown, 1997). Family therapists explore context, and the current context in which NHS funding and study leave is limited may discourage or prevent professionals from looking to extend their roles, particularly as family therapy posts are rarely found in these services. Therefore, whilst I would wholeheartedly advocate for other speech and language therapists, occupational therapists, physiotherapists, neuropsychologists, rehabilitation nurses and doctors completing the full systemic training, I realise that this is not a realistic option for everybody.

In my current NHS role in a child and adolescent mental health service, many of my colleagues have completed one, two or four years of family therapy training, and use this understanding and skill set alongside their primary training as mental health nurses, psychiatrists and psychologists. Others who have not received formal training have read systemic texts and widely acknowledge the relative influence of family relationships on mental health and vice versa, with the result that systemic thinking and practice is much more ingrained in clinical discussion and practice than I personally have encountered in 'physical' health settings, although I acknowledge that this will not reflect the practice of all neuro-rehabilitation services. Systemic formulation sessions enable formulation of the problem from the wider contexts of family and systems, rather than focusing on individual pathology.

Some have raised the question: Without professionals qualified to work in neuro-rehabilitation and family therapy, will developments in services be hindered (LarØi, 2003)? My perhaps unsurprising view is that they might be, or at least that with more confidence to explore relationships, health professionals may feel able to address some of the most meaningful issues a family can face following ABI. I believe that there would be benefit from systemic ideas being discussed more routinely in ABI rehab, and brief, basic training being provided to rehabilitation teams, either from local family therapy services, or in-house from neuropsychologists with an interest in systemic theory and practice. It may be helpful to incorporate elements of systemic formulation in team case discussions to model a systemic perspective and more deeply explore the family context. Joint working opportunities among disciplines, already frequently taken up in many neuro-rehabilitation services as part of standard practice, will continue to help reduce the fragmentation of identity that we can at times contribute to when we focus on the rehabilitation of specific skills. Joint sessions with family therapists, systemic practitioners or team members with an interest in systemic practice could extend the team's confidence in attending to systemic and relational issues, to give space to the discussion of the impact on the family of ABI and understand what support and further conversations might be helpful. To open conversations about relationships can feel daunting if we are concerned about our ability to contain the emotions that may be expressed. But by not opening up these conversations in a skilled, sensitive and supportive way, are we less well placed to explore fears, concerns, resilience and the support that might be required for a family to continue the healing journey long after ABI?

Clinical recommendations for consideration

Rehabilitation professionals can:

- Invest in the therapeutic relationship with the people we work with, considering how our professional, cultural and personal contexts influence us.
- See the aphasia as a relational, family problem rather than a problem within an individual.
- Involve family members in as much as we do as is possible for them, making the invitation clear from the start.

- Reflect on the power we have to further silence the person with aphasia, or contribute to a culture of incompetence.
- Consider the language we use with and about people, and how this can empower or disempower.
- Use problem-free talk: gain an understanding of the communication in family before the ABI, family strengths, activities, jokes . . . what characterises them other than the communication disorder?
- Promote family growth through the life cycle and resilience in the face of stressors.
- Frame the family as united against the communication disorder.
- Consider our own level of knowledge, skills, experience and confidence in working with families and relationships after ABI and seek relevant development and training opportunities as appropriate.

Neuro-rehabilitation services to consider:

- Where there might be an unmet need for family therapy or couples therapy for people accessing neuro-rehabilitation, and refer to local services as appropriate. This may involve the sharing of skills among professionals used to working with aphasia, and those who are inexperienced in working with communication disorders but experienced in systemic practice.
- Incorporating systemic formulation in team case discussion.
- Providing training opportunities for rehabilitation professionals in systemic theory and practice, whether through reading, joint working, in-service training, training from local family therapy services, or completion of systemic training to foundation, intermediate or masters level.

Considerations for further research

In addition to developing clinical work through the measures outlined above, more research is needed to understand whether increased access to conversations about relationships and increased access to psychotherapeutic approaches would translate into improved outcomes for families with aphasia. Improved outcomes may take many forms, from self-reported change in mood, to feelings of more positive family relationships, or longitudinal studies looking at the quality of long-term relationships and success of discharge. Where systemic theory and practice is already being used in ABI and aphasia services, there is a need for explicit documentation to enable further research, to identify outcomes and develop an evidence base for this work. Adapting family therapy outcome measures such as the 'SCORE-15 Index of Family Functioning and Change' (Stratton, Bland, Janes, & Lask, 2010) for families with aphasia may be a useful first step in reducing the power aphasia can have to be a barrier in accessing and evidencing this type of work.

References

AFT Website. Retrieved from www.aft.org.uk

Anderson, H., & Goolishian, H. A. (1988). Human systems as linguistic systems: Preliminary and evolving ideas about the implications for clinical theory. *Family Process*, *27*, 371–393.

Anderson, H., & Goolishian, H. A. (1992). The client is the expert: A not-knowing approach to therapy. In S. McNamee & K. J. Gergen (Eds.), *Therapy as social construction*. London: Sage Publications.

Anderson, M. I., Parmenter, T. R., & Mok, M. (2002). The relationship between neurobehavioural problems of severe Traumatic Brain Injury (TBI), family functioning and the psychological well-being of the spouse/caregiver: Path model analysis. *Brain Injury*, *16*, 743–757.

Blais, M. C., & Boisvert, J.-M. (2007). Psychological adjustment and marital satisfaction following head injury. Which critical personal characteristics should both partners develop? *Brain Injury*, *21*, 357–372.

Bowen, C. (2007). Family therapy and neuro-rehabilitation: Forging a link. *International Journal of Therapy and Rehabilitation*, *14*, 344–349.

Bowen, C., Yeates, G. N., & Palmer, S. (2010). *A relational approach to rehabilitation: Thinking about relationships after brain injury*. London: Karnac.

Burr, V. (2003). *Social constructionism* (2nd ed.). London: Routledge.

Byng, S., & Felson Duchan, J. (2005). Social model philosophies and principles: Their applications to therapies for aphasia. *Aphasiology*, *19*, 906–922.

Byng-Hall, J. (2008). The significance of children fulfilling parental roles: Implications for family therapy. *Journal of Family Therapy*, *30*, 147–162.

Cancer Research UK Race for Life Campaign (2013, February 27). 'Cancer, We're Coming to Get You' – Race for Life 2013 TV ad. (Video file). Retrieved from www.youtube.com/watch?v=GWJEmMDQXoA

Carnes, S. L., & Quinn, W. H. (2005). Family adaptation to brain injury: Coping and psychological distress. *Families, Systems, & Health*, *23*, 186–203.

Carroll, E., & Coetzer, R. (2011). Identity, grief and self-awareness after traumatic brain injury. *Neuropsychological Rehabilitation*, *21*, 289–305.

Carter, B., & McGoldrick, M. (Eds.). (1988). *The changing family life cycle: A framework for family therapy* (2nd ed.). New York: Gardner Press.

Cecchin, G. (1987). Hypothesizing, circularity, and neutrality revisited: An invitation to curiosity. *Family Process*, *26*, 405–413.

Epston, D., & Madigan, S. (1995). *From "Spy-chiatric Gaze" to communities of concern: From professional monologue to dialogue*. Retrieved from http://therapeuticconversations.com/wp-content/uploads/2017/04/Epston-Madigan-On-Leagues.pdf

Florian, V., Katz, S., & Lahav, V. (1989). Impact of traumatic brain damage on family dynamics and functioning: A review. *Brain Injury*, *3*, 219–233.

Gracey, F., Palmer, S., Rous, B., Psaila, K., Shaw, K., O'Dell, J. . . . Mohamed, S. (2008). "Feeling part of things": Personal construction of self after brain injury. *Neuropsychological Rehabilitation*, *18*, 627–650.

Hall, K., Karzmark, P., Stevens, M., Englander, J., O'Hare, P., & Wright, J. (1994). Family stressors in traumatic brain injury: A two-year follow-up. *Archives of Physical Medicine and Rehabilitation*, *75*, 876–884.

Hallett, J. D., Zasler, N. D., Maurer, P., & Cash, S. (1994). Role change after traumatic brain injury in adults. *The American Journal of Occupational Therapy*, *48*, 241–246.

Hart, A., Blincow, D., & Thomas, H. (2007). *Resilient therapy: Working with children and families*. London: Routledge.

Hartman, A. (1995). Diagrammatic assessment of family relationships. *Families in Society*, *76*, 111–122.

Headway. (2017). Website. Retrieved from www.headway.org.uk/about-brain-injury/further-information/statistics/

Herrmann, M. (1989). On the possible value of family therapy in aphasia rehabilitation. *Aphasiology*, *3*, 491–492.

Johnson, J., & McCown, W. G. (1997). *Family therapy of neurobehavioral disorders: Integrating neuropsychology and family therapy*. Oxford: Routledge.

Kagan, A. (1998). Supported conversation for adults with aphasia: Methods and resources for training conversation partners. *Aphasiology*, *12*, 816–830.

Kinsella, G., & Duffy, F. D. (1978). The spouse of the aphasic patient. In Y. Lebrun & R. Hoops (Eds.), *The management of aphasia* (pp. 26–49). Amsterdam: Swets & Zeitlinger.

Kreutzer, J. S., Gervasio, A. H., & Camplair, P. S. (1994). Primary caregivers' psychological status and family functioning after traumatic brain injury. *Brain Injury*, *8*, 197–210.

Landau, J., & Hissett, J. (2008). Mild traumatic brain injury: Impact on identity and ambiguous loss in the family. *Families, Systems, & Health*, *26*(1), 69–85.

LarØi, F. (2003). The family systems approach to treating families of persons with brain injury: A potential collaboration between family therapist and brain injury professional. *Brain Injury*, *17*, 175–187.

Leaf, L. E. (1993). Traumatic brain injury: Affecting family recovery. *Brain Injury*, *7*, 543–546.

Livingston, M. G. (1987). Head injury: The relatives' response. *Brain Injury*, *1*, 33–39.

Lock, S., Wilkinson, R., Bryan, K., Maxim, J., Edmundson, A., Bruce, C., & Moir, D. (2001). Supporting Partners of People with Aphasia in Relationships and Conversation (SPPARC). *International Journal of Language and Communication Disorders*, *36*, 25–30.

Mauss-Clum, N., & Ryan, M. (1981). Brain injury and the family. *Journal of Neuroscience Nursing*, *13*, 165–169.

Masten, A. S., Best, K. M., & Garmezy, M. (1990). Resilience and development: Contributions from the study of children who overcome adversity. *Development and Psychopathology*, *2*, 425–444.

McGoldrick, M., & Gerson, R. (1985). *Genograms in family assessment*. New York: W.W. Norton.

Meredith, K. (2012). *Exploring the process of coping in partners of people with communication disorders resulting from acquired brain injury in the early phase of neuro-rehabilitation: Experiences and reflections of a focus group. A qualitative study*. Unpublished MSc Dissertation, Institute of Psychiatry, King's College London.

Michallet, B., Tétreault, S., & Le Dorze, G. (2003). The consequences of severe aphasia on the spouses of aphasic people: A description of the adaptation process. *Aphasiology*, *17*, 835–859.

Minnes, P., Graffi, S., Nolte, M. L., Carlson, P., & Harrick, L. (2000). Coping and stress in Canadian family caregivers of persons with traumatic brain injuries. *Brain Injury*, *14*, 737–748.

Minuchin, S. (1974). *Families and family therapy*. Cambridge, MA: Harvard University Press.
Monk, G., Winslade, J., Crocket, K., & Epston, D. (Eds.). (1996). *Narrative therapy in practice: The archaeology of hope*. San Francisco, CA: Jossey-Bass.
Nichols, F., Varchevker, A., & Pring, T. (1996). Working with People with Aphasia and their Families. *Aphasiology*, *10*(8).
Norup, A., Siert, L., & Lykke Mortensen, E. (2010). Emotional distress and quality of life in relatives of patients with severe brain injury: The first month after injury. *Brain Injury*, *24*, 81–88.
Padesky, C. A., & Mooney, K. A. (2012). Strengths-based cognitive-behavioural therapy: A four-step model to build resilience. *Clinical Psychology and Psychotherapy*, *19*, 283–290.
Panting, A., & Merry, P. H. (1970). Long term rehabilitation of severe head injuries – Social and medical support for the patient's family. *Injury*, *2*, 33–37.
Perlesz, A., Kinsella, G., & Crowe, S. (1999). Impact of traumatic brain injury on the family: A critical review. *Rehabilitation Psychology*, *44*, 6–35.
Perlesz, A., Kinsella, G., & Crowe, S. (2000). Psychological distress and family satisfaction following traumatic brain injury: Injured individuals and their primary, secondary and tertiary carers. *Journal of Head Trauma Rehabilitation*, *15*, 909–929.
Pound, C., Parr, S., Lindsay, J., & Woolf, C. (2000). *Beyond aphasia*. Oxon: Winslow.
Revenson, T. A. (2003). Scenes from a marriage: Examining support, coping and gender within the context of chronic illness. In J. Suls & K. A. Wallston (Eds.), *Social psychological foundations of health and illness* (Chapter 20). Malden: Blackwell Publishing.
Rolland, J. S. (1994). In sickness and in health: The impact of illness on couples' relationships. *Journal of Marital and Family Therapy*, *20*, 327–347.
Romano, M. D. (1974). Family response to traumatic head injury. *Scandinavian Journal of Rehabilitation Medicine*, *6*, 1–4.
Rutter, M. (1999). Resilience concepts and findings: Implications for family therapy. *Journal of Family Therapy*, *21*, 119–144.
Stiell, K., & Gailey, G. (2011). Emotionally focused therapy for couples living with aphasia. In J. L. Furrow, S. M. Johnson, & B. A. Bradley (Eds.), *The emotionally focused casebook: New directions in treating couples* (Chapter 5). New York: Routledge.
Stiell, K., Naaman, S. C., & Lee, A. (2007). Couples and chronic illness: An attachment perspective and emotionally focused therapy interventions. *Journal of Systemic Therapies*, 26, 59–74.
Stratton, P. (2016). *The evidence base of family and systemic practice*. Association for Family Therapy. Merthyr Tydfil: Stephens and George Print Group.
Stratton, P., Bland, J., Janes, E., & Lask, J. (2010). Developing an indicator of family function and a practicable outcome measure for systemic family and couple therapy: The SCORE. *Journal of Family Therapy*, *32*, 232–258.
Stroke Association Website. (2019). Retrieved from https://www.stroke.org.uk/what-is-aphasia/aphasia-and-its-effects
Talking Mats Website. Retrieved from www.talkingmats.com/
Tomm, K. (1998). A question of perspective. *Journal of Marital and Family Therapy*, *24*, 409–413.
Verhaeghe, S., Defloor, T., & Grypdonck, M. (2005). Stress and coping among families of patients with traumatic brain injury: A review of the literature. *Journal of Clinical Nursing*, *14*, 1004–1012.

Wåhrborg, P. (1989). Aphasia and family therapy. *Aphasiology, 3*, 479–482.
Wåhrborg, P., & Borenstein, P. (1989). Family therapy in families with an aphasic member. *Aphasiology, 3*, 93–98.
White, M., & Epston, D. (1990). *Narrative means to therapeutic ends*. New York: Norton.
Wood, R. L., & Yurdakul, L. K. (1997). Change in relationship status following traumatic brain injury. *Brain Injury, 11*, 491–501.
World Health Organization. (2001). *The International Classification of Functioning, disability and health (ICF)*. Geneva: WHO. Retrieved from www.who.int/classifications/icf/en/
Yeates, G., Gracey, F., & Collicutt McGrath, J. (2008). A biopsychosocial deconstruction of "personality change" following acquired brain injury. *Neuropsychological Rehabilitation, 18*, 566–589.

Chapter 5

A preliminary study of "Laboratorio di Conversazione Narrativa"

Group psychotherapy supporting communication for people with aphasia

Stefano Monte, Maristella Crielesi, Marcella Di Pietro, Mariateresa Matera, Kate H. Meredith, Rossella Muò

Introduction

The term "aphasia" describes a difficulty understanding and using language, secondary to an *acquired brain injury (ABI)*. People with aphasia may have problems with speaking, understanding, writing, reading and counting. The most common cause of aphasia is stroke, but it can also be the result of traumatic brain injury or brain tumours. Difficulties with language can represent a mask, which is likely to conceal skill, intelligence and competence (Kagan & Gailey, 1993; Kagan, 1995). Aphasia can be perceived as "identity theft" (Shadden, 2005), and whilst it is easy to give a general definition of aphasia, it is harder to understand what it really means to become a person with aphasia.

Change resulting from an acquired cognitive impairment can be described as direct or indirect (Prigatano, 1986). Direct change is the direct consequence of brain injury and the neurological changes. Indirect change concerns psychological reactions of people facing the loss of capacity. The boundary between change resulting from brain injury and change associated with the reaction of the person is not always clear. Allegorically it can be said that the "gross weight" of the disability is the result of the "net weight" – cognitive impairment linked directly to the lesion – plus an additional weight (Muò, Monte, Barilari, & Di Pietro, 2010). The additional weight is significant, as it includes the emotional reaction to the loss of capacity and the relational and social consequences.

The purpose of this paper is to present a review of a psychotherapeutic group intervention at *Centro Afasia CIRP*. The Centro Afasia CIRP offers intervention based on 15 years of clinical experience. The research described in this article is distinguished by the integration of two approaches: group aphasia therapy following a social approach and psychotherapy intervention with a group analysis approach. The focus is on the process of intervention and on the research design of a psychotherapeutic group for people with aphasia. It principally describes the preliminary stages of the intervention, the research: the method, the assessment of needs, the data collection and the aims of the intervention.

Rehabilitation and psychotherapy

The aim of rehabilitation, in accordance with the philosophy widespread over the past decade by the World Health Organization (WHO), is to improve psychological well-being, independence and quality of life, as well as increasing the level of participation and social inclusion. In considering these objectives alongside complexity of need, there is a requirement for flexible interventions that are responsive to the specific nature of each individual case. The rehabilitation process should be multidisciplinary and long-term (ICF, 2001; Bioetica e Riabilitazione, 2006 webliography).

Guidelines for long-term neurological rehabilitation related to ABI emphasise the necessity of long-term management utilising different skills, rather than a short-term specific reparative intervention (National Clinical Guideline for Stroke, 2012; National Service Framework for Long-Term Neurological Conditions, 2005 webliography). Long-term rehabilitation should actively involve the caregiver and the family. This type of process includes medical interventions but is in sharp contrast to a purely medical model of care that would not be appropriate to this service provision philosophy. Understanding and acting on what ABI means for specific individuals and for their social network and family is a complex process and should be implemented across a sufficiently extended period of time (Bowen, Yeates, & Palmer, 2010).

Among the approaches to aphasia, the Social Approach is most consistent with the aims of long-term rehabilitation. The approach is thought to improve a person's communication, active participation and personal well-being at all stages of the clinical course of rehabilitation. This approach inspired ideas about the Life Participation Approach to Aphasia (LPAA) as a "social philosophy", orienting intervention, evaluation and research (LPAA Project Group, 2000; LPAA Project Group, 2001). The Social Approach was identified as an epistemological basis for organising the most appropriate interventions (Kagan, 1998a, 1998b). It is an approach focused on the active participation of the person with aphasia, who is included from the beginning to the end of the rehabilitation programme, in a health context and in a family and social interaction context (Kagan et al., 2007; Simmons-Mackie & Kagan, 2007; Simmons-Mackie et al., 2007). People's relational and communicative resources are activated by using appropriate communication supports, such as Supported Conversation for Adults with Aphasia (SCA) (Simmons-Mackie, Conklin, & Kagan, 2008). SCA is designed to help people who "know more than they can say" to express their opinions and feelings in a way that makes them feel valued and heard. The goals of SCA are to acknowledge the competence of the adult with aphasia and to help the person to reveal his or her competence (Kagan et al., 2004). Social participation is not only the aim; it is the method through which interventions are formulated, developed and implemented, from the beginning of the illness. Kagan uses the term "A-From" to underline how the final aim must be present from the first phases of care (Kagan & Simmons-Mackie, 2007). To implement a social approach to aphasia, it is essential to be able to move away from a vision of aphasia focused only on the loss of the ability.

The paradigm of impairment is orientated on deficit, and the aim of impairment-focused therapy is to improve language functions by means of procedures that stimulate specific skills. The communication-based or social-based treatment is focused on what the person is still able to do, and what is still present; it is crucial to think about the person's skills so that it is possible to use all resources available (ASHA webliography; Simmons-Mackie, 2007; Kagan, Black, Felson Duchan, Simmons-Mackie, & Square, 2001). The efficacy of group aphasia therapy has been demonstrated, with positive benefits reported (Simmons-Mackie, 2007). The involvement of people with aphasia in groups encourages communication exchange, acquisition and practice of communication strategies and the development of social relationships. The group could be considered the protected prelude, which successively extends communication skills to real-life environments (Ross, Winslow, Marchant, & Brumfitt, 2006; Elman & Bernstein-Ellis, 1999). Simmons-Mackie, Savage, and Worrall (2014) highlights:

> For example, descriptions of group conversation therapy depict conversational interaction with implicit management by the clinician, including modelling and scaffolding with natural feedback.
>
> (p. 519)

Some studies argue that for people with aphasia, the number and characteristics of activities are not as important as the opportunity to be involved (Dalemans, De Witte, Lemmens, Van Den Heuvel, & Wade, 2008). People with aphasia often feel isolated or unable to resume previous work or activities, but they may still feel active and useful. In a study that investigated social participation through the eyes of people with aphasia it emerged that:

> they wanted to feel engaged and to have a voice. They wanted to function in an ordinary way, to be respected, to know what is going on, to do things with others without being a burden, to take part in the community.
>
> (Dalemans, De Witte, Wade, & van den Heuvel, 2010, p. 540)

If the goal is to facilitate social participation, it is necessary to understand how that person reacts at the emotional and relational level. If the work is not at a deeper level, linked with the identity and with the emotions of the person, the risk will be that objectives can only be declared, without any real conditions to achieve them. Psychotherapy can be an effective tool working on complex and very specific aims, such as creating empowerment and improving the quality of life and social participation of a person who has suddenly acquired aphasia. Few articles in the literature have examined the psychotherapeutic work with people with aphasia. A review of the database (Pubmed, PsychInfo, Google Scholar) revealed few papers that met our criteria for inclusion (using keywords: "Aphasia", "group" and "psychotherapy"), other than one conducted in the US in the 1950s. Blackman (1950) is frequently cited for his psychotherapeutic group for people with aphasia. According to Blackman, the psychotherapy approach enabled people to voice emotions such as hostility and anger in a protected environment, and the group setting allowed people to develop a "stronger sense of self" (p. 156 Blackman, 1950 in Brumfitt & Sheeran, 1997). Referencing the contribution of Blackman, Brumfitt argued that the beliefs that individuals have of themselves can play an important role in rehabilitation (Brumfitt & Sheeran, 1997).

In the case of psychotherapy with couples living with aphasia (Stiell & Gailey, 2011) or ABI (Bowen et al., 2010), the goals are often to re-establish bonds and to activate self-regulatory functions. In these fields, a psychotherapist has to adjust his techniques (e.g. Emotionally Focused Couples Therapy, EFT) to the specific condition (aphasia or ABI). Stiell and Gailey (2011) suggest some strategies:

a) Psychotherapy should avoid direct questioning, because of survivor's lack of initiation. Instead, therapeutic inquiry can be supported and mediated by the signalling of a speech and language therapist.
b) There can be a great advantage in co-leading the intervention together with an expert in communication strategies, such as a speech and language therapist.
c) There is a need to create a platform to communicate adequately, involving and engaging the couple in increasing mutually accessible communication. This can be created by using the techniques in SCA or, more generally, other media such as keywords, gesture, drawing and body language.

Psychotherapy, in our clinical experience, is a tool that may help survivors and caregivers to reposition on the existential continuum interrupted by illness. For example, after the group psychotherapeutic interventions at the Centro Afasia CIRP, some people with aphasia started an integrated theatre group: *Teatro Babel* (weblink: www.facebook.com/Teatro-Babel-597685420308308/). Teatro Babel is currently composed of people with aphasia, students and volunteers. In December 2013, they made their debut in a famous theatre in Turin. One of the main characteristics of this experience is the participants' role not as "patients" induced to recite on the stage, but as "actors" projecting the scene and giving themselves a challenge. Psychotherapeutic work has been an important element, to activate an internal locus of control and mobilise available resources within the limitations related to the condition. It is fundamental for survivors to exit the role of "patient" or "sick" and re-position themselves more actively and consistently towards their own identity.

Intervention and research: "Conversazione Narrativa" workshop

The context and the research

The "Conversazione Narrativa" workshop is one of the group interventions that Centro Afasia CIRP offers. People with aphasia usually access Centro Afasia when they begin outpatient rehabilitation. They can be referred by the rehabilitation service, or they may present to the service in other ways, when their speech and language therapy is going to be completed. The average time post stroke is five to six months, but there is wide variability: from 20 days to some years. The key to accessing the interventions of the Aphasia Centre CIRP is "assessment of needs". The assessment of needs is carried out by a psychotherapist. It is divided into: first interview, clinical assessment, data collection, team meeting and delivery of a therapeutic proposal to the patient and family. People generally show different reactions to their acquired brain injury/aphasia, consistent with specific personality traits, with varied relational functioning and with the specificity of the history of life. A common element is usually the existence of an explicit demand centered on language deficits: "I cannot talk as well as before; I can't do what I did before". Emotional experience is often characterised by pain and distrust; life often appears devoid of meaning, because all seems lost and nothing more can be done. Although the patient connects the pain with the organic injury and acquired cognitive impairment, the psychotherapist also records an emotional dimension. The aim of intervention is to understand how to access this level, to support learning and transformation. Demand analysis and clinical assessment are the first steps to be able to move in this direction and strengthen therapeutic alliance. The essential transformation is to view aphasia not as a disease, but as a new way of life. The aim is to support transition from "I cannot" to a more flexible "what can I do with my limits and my resources?" It is the necessity of integration between "before" and "after", between a "healthy self" and a "sick self".

The goals of Conversazione Narrativa workshop intervention can be summarized from the collation of individual aims:

a) To improve expressive abilities, implementing communication strategies and using available communication resources;
b) To increase independence communicating, experience possibilities and increase desire to communicate with others. This goal is not only for the person in the role of making the effort to communicate, but remarkably also for the person who is trying to understand;
c) To increase psychological well-being by promoting self-esteem and awareness of resources in relation to limits.

Method

The word "laboratorio" means "workshop". It is not a closed, sterile place; it is not performativity or training; it is a forge where everyone (therapists and patients) actively participate in the achievement of explicit objectives, aimed at social participation. The term "conversazione" ("conversation") represents a natural and social kind of communication; it is shared and non-directive. The term "narrativa" ("narrative") means the opportunity to share relevant stories. "Laboratorio Conversazione Narrativa" is a psychotherapeutic intervention group, proposed as a therapeutic opportunity to people whose individual needs are suited to the nature of the intervention. There is a coordination of professionals' input: a psychotherapist (group-analytic therapist) and a speech and language therapist skilled in verbal communication strategies. The professionals do not lead but facilitate, to enable each person to use their resources in a circular communication.

The project is structured in the following phases:

1 Individual phase: preparing for the group;
2 Group intervention;
3 Individual stage: evaluation of change and retest (T1).

The overall duration of the intervention is approximately 16 months. The individual phase can be of variable length, depending on the individual case. Group intervention lasts approximately eight months, and the completion date is discussed during the first meeting. The individual meetings occur once a week, for approximately 50 minutes. The group meetings are held once a week, for approximately 1 hour and 30 minutes.

The investigation of the clinical process and effectiveness was based on clinical evaluation and clinical observation. Co-conduction of the group and weekly comparison between other psychotherapists of the centre was a source of further learning.

The six identified participants had a homogeneous level of aphasia (severity and type, understanding was not compromised). The intervention is not suitable for people who have disorders of consciousness, thought or cognitive impairment of higher cortical functions in addition to language issues, assessed by neuropsychological tests and neurological examination.

1 INDIVIDUAL PHASE: PREPARING FOR THE GROUP

In the individual phase, following the assessment of needs, all participants are tested before intervention (T0) and after intervention (T1). This phase is preliminary to work in groups. It uses the information obtained during the stage of the analysis of needs to specify the personal goals of the patient linked with group intervention. Personal goals vary from person to person. Each person is presented with different expectations, including improving language and communication, managing the emotions that interfere with communication, intending to be understandable to others and also establishing friendships.

The choice of specific evaluation measures provides the following information:

Language, communication, pragmatic abilities and evaluation of emotion tests

AAT – Aachner Aphasie Test (Luzzatti, De Bleser, & Willmes, 1991)
Assesses spontaneous speech, repetition, written language, naming and comprehension (Gialannella, 2011)

I-ASHA-FACS – Functional Assessment of Communication Skills for Adults (Muò, et al. 2015)
A measure of basic functional skills that are common to the majority of individuals regardless of age, gender, socioeconomic status, educational/vocational status or cultural diversity (Muò et al., 2015)

ASHA NOMS and **rating scale of pragmatic abilities** (ASHA webliography)
A scale to stage pragmatic abilities in persons with communication disorders

VAMS – Visual Analogue Mood Scales (Stern, 1999)
A self-report mood test, developed specifically for neurologically impaired patients in general and people with aphasia in particular. This scale assesses eight mood states: sad, happy, tense, afraid, tired, energetic, confused and angry (Stern, 1999)

Caregivers' Tests

SADQ-10-Stroke Aphasic Depression Questionnaire (Sutcliffe & Lincoln, 1998)
A 10-item questionnaire that reflects observable behaviour associated with low mood, indirectly reported by the caregiver

CBI – Caregiver Burden Inventory (Novak Guest C., 1989)
A 24-item, multi-dimensional questionnaire measuring caregiver burden with five subscales:
(a) Time dependence; (b) Developmental; (c) Behaviour; (d) Physical burden; (e) Social burden; (f) Emotional burden

BDI – Beck Depression Inventory (Beck, Ward, Mendelson, Mock, & Erbaugh, 1961)
A 21-question, multiple-choice, self-report inventory, used to measures caregiver's mood

---

Measurements are also taken of the electrical activity of the brain in a spontaneous situation (Brain Mapping QEEG) and in an event-related situation (ERP), to record the changes on a neurological level before (T0) and after (T1) intervention. The N400 and P300 have been investigated. N400 is part of the normal electrophysiological brain response towards any other meaningful (or potentially meaningful) verbal stimuli (Kutas, 2000). P300 reflects the process of assessment and categorization of a stimulus.

Evaluation methods also include recording a video and using a Likert scale (from 1–10, not standardized) to record the perception of aphasia burden in daily life.

At the end of this stage, it was possible to finalize the project of the intervention group. The psychotherapist could identify the general purposes and identify the next group stages' parameters.

General aims were:

1 Create a communication platform that encourages use of expertise and promotes participation in the group.
2 Address the difficulties associated with limits of communication: make it less "deficit heavy", facilitate the experience of "you can" rather than on "you cannot anymore".
3 Identify communication strategies: while the group works, the speech and language therapist uses her skills to identify and point out possible strategies.

2 GROUP INTERVENTION

The group constitutes a social network to connect the clinical/rehabilitation context (secondary social network) to a personal context (primary social network) (Fasolo et al., 2003). It is not only rehabilitation practice, but also as close a context as possible to the social dimension (Fasolo, Ambrosiano, & Cordioli, 2004). The *Operative Group* is a theoretical framework within which to place the nature of the intervention. The operative group was born in the early forties in a psychiatric context; its aim was to increase the work of the healthcare team, working on the skills of the staff and of the less severe patients. Pichon-Rivière defines it as a group technique that is centered on a task. Usually the explicit goal is learning, healing, communication or coping and empowerment. This task also has an implicit aspect, associated with the difficulties that arise in its implementation as a stereotype that impedes learning and communication, thus acting as an obstacle to any progress or change (Pichon-Rivière, 1971, 1978, 1981). This is similar to the definition of group analysis as a method and a technique based on the dynamics of the group (Tubert-Oklander & Hernandez de Tubert, 2004). Group analysis is not psychoanalysis of individuals in a group; it is a therapy in the group, of the group and by the group. Intra-psychic processes are seen as interacting within the mental matrix of the group as a whole (Foulkes, 1986). However, the distinction of the operative group is the common task that becomes one of the main organizers of its dynamics (Tubert-Oklander & Hernandez de Tubert, 2004). The operative group is a group of people linked by a common goal, which they try to achieve by working as a team. The problems and the difficulties arising are dealt by the group gradually (Bleger, 2011). The group facilitator is a coordinator or a co-thinker. He coordinates the efforts of the participants and helps them to think, by thinking with them (Tubert-Oklander & Hernandez de Tubert, 2004). The task of the operative group is generally associated with learning. Learning is not intended as a technical teaching or as a transferring by those who know to those who do not know. Learning is a transformation process and includes the experience of "do not know" as a basis. This requires the ability to think beyond stereotypes

(Bleger, 2011). For Bion, the development of thinking is based on issues linked with absence. In fact, an appropriate function of thinking makes absence representable rather than a "nameless dread", but it requires one to tolerate uncertainty (Bion, 1962). The work on the task of the operative group is not a spontaneous activity for its members, but it is difficult and emotionally arduous. The psychotherapist facilitator of the group is a coordinator; rather than being an expert teaching something, his role is to facilitate the working group on the task (Bleger, 2011). His initial aim is to create an adequate setting for the group's operation. Then it is to understand, and make understandable, the defensive blocks that cause resistance to change and prevent learning (Pichon-Rivière, 1971, 1978).

In terms of group dynamics, both the psychotherapist and speech and language therapist are more facilitators than leaders. Both are members of an operative group, bringing their specific expertise as resources for the team. The psychotherapist uses his expertise to promote the birth of circular communication. He can also facilitate the elaboration of difficulties that will arise while the group is working on communication. This level, as mentioned earlier, is not always explicit and thus it may hinder the work. At the same time, learning how to deal with such difficulties is considered to be very important in the daily life of a person with aphasia. The speech and language therapist uses her knowledge to focus on communication. She is active in proposing a communication platform that is able to take adequate account of the linguistic deficit, but also to allow everyone to participate. We hypothesize that this plays an important role in a meta-level communication: the identification of strategies from emerging conversational content.

Both facilitators are trained in use of supportive conversation techniques according to the principles of shared LPAA techniques, such as SCA.

The facilitators suggest some key phases for the group:

1 Initial stage: the therapeutic contract;
2 A knowledge phase: the management may be more active;
3 Activation of a communication network, the measure of participation;
4 The group tries to reflect and reason about communication;
5 Group learning strategies.

The contract marks the beginning of the operative group; other phases are not sequential, but they are group functioning levels. These levels can also give indications of the emotional difficulties associated with the task. If the group were paralyzed by anxieties and difficulties, its communication would tend to be basic and dependent on facilitators.

The therapist proposes a therapeutic contract during the first group meeting by defining the purpose of the group (the task) in a clear and shared way, and to share the setting of other parameters. The contract has the function of a compass, to give useful references in the most difficult moments. It is an explicit part of the job so it must be clear and shared.

The therapist proposes the following points to the group:

1. Presentation and explanation of individual expectations;
2. Summary of individual expectations and framing of a clear and shared task;
3. Date of completion of the work, duration of each meeting, rules to be shared for the protection of the group. These are referred to as "common standards"; however, it is important to make them explicit (e.g. punctuality, attendance, notice in the event of a delay or absence);
4. The core characteristic of the group: the conversation. Conversation is understood as communicative activities based on participation, and on personal tales;
5. The group is proposed as the place in which it is possible to develop the relevant issues.

3 INDIVIDUAL STAGE: EVALUATION OF CHANGE AND RETEST (T1)

The end of the group work is followed by two or three individual interviews with the person with aphasia and their caregiver, moving from the group dimension to a personal and family dimension.

These interviews review the personal goals identified in the individual phase, and the team goals.

The interviews enable reflection and an evaluation of the group work, including questions such as:

1. How did you feel?
2. Have there been important learning moments or events?
3. How was the work, the expectations and the task?

This step completes the clinical assessment and returns to the individual treatment plan. Psychological, relational and communicative aspects are assessed with the patient and family. Rehabilitation plans may be revised or concluded. Usually, when the patient finishes their rehabilitation at the CIRP center, follow-ups will be expected over time. In the final individual stage, the person is tested again.

Discussion

This study is focused on a psychotherapeutic group intervention for people with aphasia. The aim is the explanation of the parameters orienting intervention and research. The goal is to clarify "what we do" and "how we do it". Data of T0 and T1 are not presented in this article; a study of statistical quantitative data is in progress. However, we can propose some reflections as a work in progress, based on the present clinical observations.

"Belongingness" (or the sense of group belonging) was active from the first steps, and it has facilitated the participation of the members from the beginning. The careful individual preparation for the group and the common condition of aphasia has enabled the establishment of belongingness. The group setting and tasks immediately activate a *new role for the clients*; they are no longer only a person with aphasia with problems in communicative output; they are also a person skilled in understanding and helping others to communicate. It is as if taking part in the group could slowly awaken a person's sleeping cognitive and social skills. This is an important therapeutic function for the group, as well as a pattern of individual empowerment. Initially, spontaneous communication takes place in a linear way and is dependent on the facilitator, with each client seeking facilitation for himself. In this phase, the group was like a sum of people with aphasia who were focused on their linguistic difficulties. However, the transition to a more interactive modality of communication is relatively swift – clients begin to interact and to participate as early as the fourth meeting.

A qualitative clinical judgement is that there has been a *general implementation of self-esteem and empowerment* for the participants. These qualities can be linked to some of the learning shared by the people with aphasia:

- A greater awareness of limits and of resources;
- The acceptance of the condition of "aphasic people, but not only aphasic";
- The attenuation of the emotions for the failure of communication that interfere with communicative initiative and motivation.

A general development in self-perception has also been noted. *Self-representation where the primary identifier was "being disabled" has given way to the awareness of relational and social possibilities*. This may be linked with these observations:

- Desire and ability to participate in new social and relational activities;
- Increased desire to communicate, which is reflected in greater initiative in the conversation;
- Greater chance of re-positioning of role in relation to its reference social network.

The confrontation with members of the group allows the person with aphasia to re-evaluate their perception of disability. In the Conversazione Narrativa workshop, each participant who actively supported peer communication returned to him/herself a feeling of usefulness and value. During the group, it was possible to bring out *new, more adaptive coping strategies focused on emotions*. The participants could recognize and manage emotions of frustration, helplessness, shame, anger and sadness. The disturbing emotions such as anticipatory anxiety, which worsened the linguistic performance and forms of reactive depression, which induced withdrawal, have eased. Also for these reasons, the communicative initiative of the participants may be extended to the context of real life. Concretely, the person is going to increase social participation.

In addition, the *contribution of the caregiver* has been as important in determining the outcome of the intervention. The contribution of the caregiver has allowed another point of view regarding changes, and feedback about emotional management skills and the communication level of the person with aphasia. Furthermore, the relative can describe their perception in terms of the degree of dependence in everyday life. In this research, caregivers reported feeling less burden, as the person with aphasia gained greater confidence in their communicative ability and avoided fewer communicative situations. People with aphasia participated more in communicative situations, with implications for their quality of life and that of their families.

In addition to these clinical considerations, the preliminary analysis of ERP data shows increased amplitude and reduced latency of the N400 that is supposed to indicate *a greater speed and accuracy when drawing up verbal information.* Based on the results of the intervention, there is an impact on quality, understood as accuracy and naming speed. The same trend also concerns the P300 ERP wave. The P300 allows us to understand how effective the cognitive system is in recognising a stimulus.

Conclusion

At this point of the study seems to emerge the different representation of itself, especially with regard to the subjective experience of aphasia, with real relapses in the relational and social sphere of the participants.

The data analysis is not yet concluded, but once this has occurred it will allow evaluation of the effectiveness of the intervention and help provide a possible direction for future research.

It will be necessary to assess the progress of communicative and psychological learning beyond the group and how learning may change over time. It will be useful to schedule a follow-up one year after the end of the work.

Many other variables require evaluation, including feedback on the results in relation to the assumptions, the different therapeutic functions linked with the facilitation and with the group process, the trend of communication throughout all the interventions, and the relationship between all these elements. Specifically, group dynamics will need to be assessed, considering co-conduction and group therapeutic factors (group climate, therapeutic alliance, empathy, cohesion, etc.). It is necessary to consider the complexity of administering non-analogic tests for the evaluation of the process and outcome of psychotherapy intervention. It will also be important to study the relationship of all these elements together: the results and the clinical and communicative sphere process.

References

Beck, A.T., Ward, C.H., Mendelson, M., Mock, J., & Erbaugh, J. (1961). An inventory for measuring depression. *Archives of General Psychiatry*, *4*, 561–571.

Bion, W. R. (1962). *Learning from experience*. London: Karnac Books.

Blackman, N. M. D. (1950, February). Group psychotherapy with aphasics. *Journal of Nervous & Mental Disease*, *111*(2), 154–163.

Bleger, J. (2011). *Psicoigiene e Psicologia Istituzionale*. Molfetta, BA: La Merdiana.

Bowen, C., Yeates, G. N., & Palmer, S. (2010). *A relational approach to rehabilitation: Thinking about relationships after brain injury*. London: Karnac.

Brumfitt, S. M., & Sheeran, P. (1997). An evaluation of short-term group therapy for people with aphasia. *Disability and Rehabilitation*, *19*(6), 221–230.

Comitato Nazionale per la Bioetica, Presidenza del Consiglio dei Ministri. (2006, March 17). *Bioetica e Riabilitazione*. Retrieved from http://bioetica.governo.it/it/in webliography

Dalemans, R. J. P., De Witte, L. P., Lemmens, J., van den Heuvel, W. J., & Wade, D. T. (2008). Measures for rating social participation in people with aphasia: A systematic review. *Clinical Rehabilitation*, *22*(6), 542–555.

Dalemans, R. J. P., De Witte, L. P., Wade, D., & van den Heuvel, W. J. (2010, September–October). Social participation through the eyes of people with aphasia. *International Journal of Language & Communication Disorders*, *45*(5), 537–550.

Elman, R., & Bernstein-Ellis, E. (1999). The efficacy of group communication treatment in adults with chronic aphasia. *Journal of Speech, Language, and Hearing Research*, *42*, 411–419.

Fasolo, F., Ambrosiano, I., & Cordioli, A. (2004). Reti sociali e gruppi terapeutici: teorie e tecniche biologiche cruciali per la psichiatria pubblica. *Narrare il Gruppo. Prospettive cliniche e Sociali*, *1*, 31–52.

Fasolo, F., Tirelli, M., Batocchio, B., Berton, A., Ferlin, M., Gallini, P. . . . Tedeschi, D. (2003). Il gruppo terapeutico come rete sociale "intermedia" e la Carta di Rete come tecnica specifica di "mind-imaging". *Psichiatriagenerale e dell'etàevolutiva*, *40*(2).

Foulkes, S. H. (1986). *Group-analytic psychotherapy: Method and principles*. London: Maresfield Library.

Gialannella, B. (2011). Aphasia assessment and functional outcome prediction in patients with aphasia after stroke. *Journal of Neurology*, *258*, 343–349.

Kagan, A. (1995). Revealing the competence of aphasic adults through conversation: A challenge to health professionals. *Topics in Stroke Rehabilitation*, *2*(1), 15–28.

Kagan, A. (1998a). Supported conversation for adults with aphasia: Methods and resources for training conversation partners. *Aphasiology*, *12*(9), 816–830.

Kagan, A. (1998b). Philosophical, practical and evaluative issues associated with Supported Conversation for Adults with Aphasia: A reply. *Aphasiology*, *12*(9), 851–864.

Kagan, A., Black, S., Felson Duchan, J., Simmons-Mackie, N., & Square, P. (2001). Training volunteers as conversation partners using "Supported Conversation for Adults with Aphasia" (SCA): A controlled trial. *Journal of Speech, Language, and Hearing Research*, *44*(3), 624–638.

Kagan, A., & Gailey, G. (1993). Functional is not enough: Training conversation partners for aphasic adults. In A. Holland & M. Forbes (Eds.), *Aphasia treatment: World perspectives* (pp. 199–215). San Diego, CA: Singular.

Kagan, A., & Simmons-Mackie, N. (2007). Beginning with the end. Outcome-driven assessment and intervention with life participation in mind. *Topics in Language Disorders*, *27*(4), 309–317.

Kagan, A., Simmons-Mackie, N., Rowland, A., Huijbregts, M., Shumway, E., McEwen, S. . . . Sharp, S. (2007). Counting what counts: A framework for capturing real-life outcomes of aphasia intervention. *Aphasiology*, 1–23.

Kagan, A., Winckel, J., Black, S., Felson Duchan, J., Simmons-Mackie, N., & Square, P. (2004). A set of observational measures for rating support and participation in conversation between adults with aphasia and their conversation partners. *Stroke Rehabilitation, 11*(1), 67–83.

Kaplan-Solms, K., & Solms, M. (2000). *Clinical studies in neuro-psychoanalysis: Introduction to a depth neuropsychology*. London: Karnac.

Kutas, M., & Federmeier, K. D. (2000). Electrophysiology reveals semantic memory use in language comprehension. *Trends in Cognitive Science, 4*(12), 463–470.

LPAA Project Group (Chapey, R., Duchan, J. F., Elman, R. J., Garcia, L. J., Kagan, A., Lyon, J., & Simmons, M. N.). (2000). Life participation approach to aphasia: A statement of values for the future. *ASHA Leader, 5*(3), 4–6. Retrieved from www.asha.org/public/speech/disorders/LPAA.htm.

LPAA Project Group (Chapey, R., Duchan, J. F., Elman, R. J., Garcia, L. J., Kagan, A., Lyon, J., & Simmons, M. N.). (2001). Life participation approach to aphasia. In R. Chapey (Ed.), *Language intervention strategies in aphasia and related neurogenic communication disorders* (4th ed., pp. 235–245). Baltimore, MD: Lippincott, Williams & Wilkins.

Luzzatti, C., De Bleser, R., & Willmes, K. (1991). *Aachener Afasie Test (AAT)*. Firenze: Organizzazioni Sociali.

Muò, R., Cancialosi, P., Galimberti, L., Cacciola, B., Gilardone, M., & Schindler, A. (2015). Validation of the Italian version of the American Speech-Language and Hearing Association – Functional Assessment of Communication Skills for adults (I-ASHA-FACS). *Aphasiology, 29*(9), 1110–1130.

Muò, R., Monte, S., Barilari, G., & Di Pietro, M. (2010). Riabilitazione nella fase degli esiti. *ActaPhonLat, 32*(1–2), 272–288.

Novak, M., & Guest C. (1989, December). Application of a multidimensional caregiver burden inventory. *The Gerontologist, 29*(6), 798–803.

Pichon-Rivière, E. (1971). *Del psicoanálisis a la psicología social* (Tomos I y II). Buenos Aires: Galerna.

Pichon-Rivière, E. (1978). *Elprocesocreador. Del psicoanálisis a la psicología social (III)*. Buenos Aires: NuevaVisión.

Pichon-Rivière, E. (1981). *Elprocesogrupal. Del psicoanálisis a la psicología social (I)*. Buenos Aires: Nueva Visión.

Prigatano, G. P. (1986). *Neuropsychological rehabilitation after brain injury*. Baltimore: Johns Hopkins University Press.

Royal College of Physicians. (2012). *Nacional clinical guideline for stroke* (4th ed.). London: Royal College of Physicians 11 St Andrews Place Regent's Park NW1 4LE.

Ross, A., Winslow, I., Marchant, P., & Brumfitt, S. (2006). Evaluation of communication, life participation and psychological well-being in chronic aphasia: The influence of group intervention. *Aphasiology, 20*(5), 427–448.

Shadden, B. B. (2005). Aphasia as identity theft. Theory and practice. *Aphasiology, 19*, 211–223.

Simmons-Mackie, N., Conklin, J., & Kagan, A. (2008). Think tank deliberates future directions for the social approach to aphasia. *Perspectives on Neurophysiology and Neurogenic Speech and Language Disorders, 18*, 24–32.

Simmons-Mackie, N., & Kagan, A. (2007). Application of the ICF in aphasia. *Seminars in Speech and Language, 28*(4), 244–253.

Simmons-Mackie, N., Kagan, A., O'Neill Christie, C., Huijbregts, M., McEwen, S., & Willems, J. (2007). Communicative access and decision making for people with aphasia: Implementing sustainable health care systems change. *Aphasiology, 27*(1), 39–66.

Simmons-Mackie, N., Savage, M. C., & Worrall, L. (2014, September–October). Conversation therapy for aphasia: A qualitative review of the literature. *International Journal of Language & Communication Disorders*, *49*(5), 511–526.
Stern, A. R. (1999). Assessment of mood states in Aphasia. *Seminars in Speech and Language*, *20*(1), 33–50.
Stiell, K., & Gailey, G. (2011). Emotionally focused therapy (E.F.T.) for couples living with aphasia. In J. L. Furrow, S. M. Johnson, & B. A. Bradley (Eds.), *The emotionally focused casebook: New directions in treating couples*. New York: Routledge Taylor & Francis Group.
Tubert-Oklander, J., & Hernandez de Tubert, R. (2004). *Operative groups: The Latin-American approach to group analysis*. London: Jessica Kingsley.
World Health Organization. (2001). *International Classification of Functioning, disability and health (ICF)*. Geneva: WHO. Retrieved from www.who.int/classifications/icf/en/

Webography

www.asha.org/
www.asha.org/PRPSpecificTopic.aspx?folderid=8589934663&section=Treatment
www.facebook.com/Teatro-Babel-597685420308308/
http://bioetica.governo.it/it/
https://www.gov.uk/government/publications/quality-standards-for-supporting-people-with-long-term-conditions

Chapter 6

Structured narrative therapy for children with acquired brain injury and severe communication difficulties

Alison Perkins

If left unchallenged, an acquired brain injury (ABI) imposes its own preferred narrative of omnipotence and a desire to invade all boundaries. Unsatisfied with changing the child's experience of the world, ABI reaches further to change the children's perception of how they individually think and feel in response to the world (Wolfe et al., 2014).

Consequently, ABI has an unparalleled power to derail the developmental process behind the injured children's concept of who they are and their own identities (Lloyd et al., 2015). Rehabilitation interventions need to attend to children's developing identity as well as their functional skills (Ownsworth & Clare, 2006).

My own workplace, the Children's Trust, provides residential multidisciplinary rehabilitation for children and teenagers in the months following a severe ABI. In this setting I have gradually developed a structured narrative intervention which invites the injured child into family communication and education over his or her brain injury and needs whilst also attending to the child's identity. I have used it with young people aged 7 to 19 years. The therapy is a structured adaptation of a narrative intervention developed by Michael White (White, 2005) for children who have experienced extreme trauma and loss. It uses the protection and positive identity construction offered by White's narrative intervention within a structured approach to accommodate the child's acquired cognitive difficulties.

Through this structured narrative approach, the injured children take control in learning about their situation and in communicating over this with their families. Usually, I offer structured narrative therapy (SNT) to children with sufficient physical, sensory and communication skills to direct and control their own exploration into their situation. This work is described elsewhere (Perkins, 2015), along with an illustrative practice example. This chapter gives a brief overview of SNT. It then describes how we adapted the SNT for Theo, a child whose ABI resulted in severe communication and physical difficulties that reduced his control.

Practical application of structured narrative therapy

SNT is a gentle, child-centred approach that helps a child gain information about their situation and acquired needs, and to establish communication with their family over these. The intervention acknowledges the potential threat from the ABI on the child's developing identity (Gracey, Evans, & Malley, 2009) and aims to set a more positive trajectory for this. Within the therapy, the child creates an autobiographical document that represents their past, present and future. Initially, the child and therapist create a document of several empty chapters covering the child's lifespan in chronological sequence. The child knows that they own this document and will take it away with them when therapy ends. The child then takes full control in building the autobiographical contents, dipping in and out of different chapters as they wish.

Documents often contain photographs, pictures and the child's dictated text. It can be built using a computer; however, a paper copy is often utilised to maximise the child's physical control over how it is accessed and shared. The child builds their autobiographical story, choosing events and relationships that are important to them. Children often start by building their early lives, using these as 'safe places to stand' (White, 2005) at a distance to their recent injury. As they work together, the therapist listens out for skills and resources that the child has used in the past. Resources that resonate with the child are thickened and woven through their past to create positive stories of skill and mastery.

Children often use these stories as the springboard by which to explore the recent events surrounding their injury, rehabilitation and future. The stories become subordinate stories of skills and mastery by which the child has managed adversity (White, 2005). Most children invite family members into sessions to witness their autobiographical document and to work on sections together. During these shared sessions, the therapist models how to maximise the child's control. The therapist constantly monitors the child's attachment to their document, and reattends to its safety, accessibility and positive stories if the child starts to disengage. When undertaking SNT with a child, parallel work is always carried out with family members before, during and after the narrative work. The focus of this family work is to ensure that they understand the model and therapeutic approach, to prepare them for their important role within the therapy, to reflect on their experience of the therapy and to monitor the emotional regulation of the family and child since this is foundational to the narrative work.

Rationale for using SNT

It is well documented that individuals with an ABI need to gain insight into their acquired needs to improve their long-term independence and quality of life (Caplan et al., 2016). Within paediatric ABI, all goals and interventions should be selected according to a developmental framework that considers the child's existing capacities, as illustrated by the Paediatric Neurocognitive Intervention (PNI), which guides the selection of neurocognitive interventions (Limond et al., 2014). I use a similar developmental framework (Figure 6.1) to guide my selection of interventions over helping the child develop insight into their injury and needs. My framework is provisional and references the PNI (Limond et al., 2014), as well as neuropsychological models of insight (Gracey, Longworth, & Psaila, 2016),

HIGHEST RESOURCES

Level 5: Child gains independence in rehabilitation: anticipation of needs, flexible and proactive strategies

- Child starts to adapt own strategies to suit current or anticipated context, including seeking social support and advocating for own needs
- Child starts to show anticipatory self-awareness of difficulties and learns to apply pre-emptive strategies
- Child spontaneously shows emergent awareness of needs & learns to apply key strategies with support
- Family communication and problem solving over difficulties becomes flexible
- Family roles become more flexible and adaptive to increased independence of injured child

Level4: Child gains intellectual & emergent awareness of situation, acquired needs, strategies

- ☐ Child fully oriented to journey (level 2), & can tolerate reflection of strengths, acquired needs, coping strategies, problem solving
- ☐ Child tolerates or requests extended, explicit brain injury education
- ☐ Child has sufficient emotional & metacognitive skills to benefit from Cognitive Behaviour Therapy
- ☐ Child can participate in the creation of information for others over situation & needs (eg family, school, peers)
- ☐ Child starts to shows emergent self-awareness of needs within daily routine and intensive practice of skills
- ☐ Family have made meaning of events surrounding ABI, family communication over situation has become open and emotionally authentic, able to look to future

Level 3: Child undertakes Intensive Practice of core skills

- Child tolerates intensive practice of key strategies & skills (physical, self-help, cognitive, educational) delivered across contexts by teachers, therapists or parents
- Child understands their need for intensive practice of key rehabilitation strategies (this will differ across physical, educational, cognitive, social domains)
- Child has understanding of 'practice - improvement' link
- Family communication & problem solving over situation becomes routine and involves injured child

Level 2: Child learns Key Information & Daily Rehabilitation Skills

- Child experiences daily rehabilitation routine - Fully supported, all contexts, natural supports
- Child gains cohesive, factual understanding of their situation (injury, rehabilitation needs, strategies, & discharge plans) as foundation for intellectual self-awareness
- Parent - child communication over situation and needs is established, including simple problem solving & planning
- Child has sufficient tolerance of threat to identity implied by daily rehabilitation & use of aids

Level 1: Child experiencing significant emotional dysregulation due to:

- ☐ Acute emotional distress (e.g. acute identity threat, mental health symptoms, poor advocacy, poor attachments, very poor quality of life)
- ☐ Acute family stressors causing systemic dysregulation
- ☐ Child is uninformed over situation or daily routine due to poor availability of information, or poor access due to sensory or cognitive impairments
- ☐ Acute behavioural dysregulation (challenging behaviour, self-harm)
- ☐ Acute medical needs (e.g. acute fatigue, epilepsy, pain, muscle tone invasive medical procedures)
- ☐ Cognitive: post traumatic amnesia, low arousal, low awareness

LOWEST RESOURCES

Figure 6.1 Provisional developmental model of capacities required to develop insight

Krasny-Pacini et al. 2015), developmental models of self-awareness (Harter, 2012) and systemic family resources for managing adversity (Walsh, 2012). It guides me when to offer SNT. Similar to the PNI, the table represents a hierarchical pyramid of the child's capacities as these increase from lower levels to higher levels. It is, therefore, intended to be read from base to tip, to show this developmental progression.

Within this developmental framework, SNT is a Level 2 intervention. It aims to help a child gain factual information about his or her situation and to safely communicate with the child's family over this. SNT is selected once the child gains sufficient emotional and behavioural regulation through the use of Level 1 interventions, such as orientation, positive behaviour support, regulatory family work, medical interventions, environmental interventions or therapeutic interventions offering non-directive containment. SNT can pave the way towards higher level interventions, such as family problem-solving interventions (Wade & Hung, 2015), structured family interventions (Gan, Gargaro, Kreutzer, Boschen, & Wright, 2010) or cognitive behaviour therapy (Waldron, Casserly, & O'Sullivan, 2013).

The aims of SNT

This hierarchical framework defines the following aims for structured narrative therapy:

- For the child to gain information over his or her injury and rehabilitation needs. The level of detail is determined by the child to avoid emotional dysregulation.
- To establish communication between child and his or her family over the child's acquired needs, in which the child holds an empowered and central position. This can be expanded to include the child's teachers and peers, whilst preventing the child from becoming marginalised from this communication (Yeates, Henwood, Gracey, & Evans, 2007).

Protecting the child's identity to manage the implicit threat within rehabilitation and to pave the way towards positive identity development as child matures. The therapy takes a narrative, post-modernist position on identity construction that proposes multiple representations of self-development in different contexts. It assumes that some self-representations have the flexibility and durability to exist across time and contexts to give an authentic 'essence of self' (Harter, 2012).

The ABI has propelled the child into a context of disempowerment and dependency. This implicates a dominant story involving self-representations of 'passivity', damage' and 'needing to be fixed by others'. SNT invites the child to look across their past and to select skills and resources that feel important and re-emerge across different times and contexts. The child and therapist thicken these authentic self-representations into positive stories of identity, giving them detail and highlighting their endurance and flexibility.

The document then invites the child to trace how they have used these skills and resources to manage their recent injury and early recovery. By doing this, the final document presents the development of positive and authentic self-representations which have the endurance and flexibility to be used in the face of acute adversity. The final document also symbolises the child's empowered decision to explore some of the recent events that threaten their identity.

Most children become very proud of their document. This is why empowering the child to take control over the discovery and discussion about their situation is so critical to SNT. For this reason, the therapist usually works with the child first to establish his or her control and then expands outwards to include the family.

How to establish Theo's control, whose ABI resulted in severe communication difficulties, posed a lot of challenges as described next.

Adapting SNT for Theo: a practice example

Theo, aged 11, lived at home with his parents and two younger siblings, Daniel and Emily. He was academic, gentle natured and slightly shy; however, made some close friends over his first term at secondary school. At Christmas, he became unwell, lost consciousness and was admitted to hospital with meningoencephalitis, which caused a severe brain injury. Investigations showed widespread inflammation throughout his brain, involving both grey matter and the white connective tissue. Theo remained in hospital for three months. He then stayed in our rehabilitation unit for six months with his mother, Grace, before returning to live at home.

On his arrival to us, Theo was wheelchair bound and unable to communicate or handle objects functionally. As the inflammation in his brain reduced, his gross motor skills recovered such that he could walk, run and climb. Certain contexts became meaningful: he could listen to a storybook, ride a tricycle and eat a meal. Outside of these settings, he lost his functional skills and was drawn into repetitive sensory responses. He understood some spoken language but could not communicate his needs, which frequently led to acute distress. We hypothesised that he experienced highly fragmented cognition, reflecting widespread disruption to his brain circuitry. I worked with Grace and the team to reduce his agitation, develop meaningful contexts to promote his skills and optimise his communication.

Six weeks before discharge, we observed Theo's attention and processing improve, although his motor and verbal apraxia continued to preclude formal assessments. He demonstrated more cognitive skills in a wider range of contexts. He could now sit and attend in class and show recognition of numbers and text using simple multiple choice. He could understand and retain simple spoken language. He could read, understand and retain simple passages of text, one or two sentences in length. He also started to join in reciprocal social games, such as hide-and-seek. He started to approach others to meet his needs. He remained unable to speak but if calm, he could indicate yes or no to simple questions using body language. He started to use a simple press button communication device. He remained unable to use everyday objects functionally; for example, he could not turn the pages of a book, use a pen, point to named objects or pictures or build with Lego. Consequently, he required full support during his personal care.

Grace celebrated this sudden improvement in Theo's skills, but it prompted her to consider Theo's understanding of his situation. She had occasionally given a short explanation of his illness to orient him to our setting but could never tell whether he found it meaningful. She stopped altogether when his cognition suddenly improved, since her own experience of learning about his illness had been traumatic. She wanted Theo to have an understanding of his illness and needs, and to advocate within his discharge plans. However, she was unsure what he wanted to know, and Theo was unable to spontaneously ask. I negotiated with Grace that maximising Theo's control in learning about his situation would show us what he wanted to know and prevent us from overwhelming his coping strategies.

Grace set the following two goals within a Goal Attainment Scaling (GAS) approach:

Goal 1: To provide Theo with a means by which he can initiate and control what he learns about his situation

Goal 2: To increase Theo's knowledge about his illness, his rehabilitation and discharge home

Theo's improved skills had helped him gain emotional regulation. This allowed me to offer SNT to achieve Grace's goals. I explained the usual process in which the child builds an autobiographical document to represent their skills and resources, and then explores how they used these resources to survive their experience of brain injury. This approach appealed to Grace, and we planned how to adapt the SNT to accommodate Theo's cognitive, communication and functional difficulties.

We decided to offer Theo an initial version of his autobiography. This would show him our offer to learn more about his situation, create a reading context that he understood and support his cognition. We would also offer enjoyable games to give him the option to refuse his autobiography. Theo would then direct how his autobiography developed. We created the initial autobiography with the guidance of Theo's team, using clear photographs and simple text that he could process, reason with and retain with repetition.

We presented his story in a predictable, chronological sequence of colour coded chapters: 'Theo and his family', 'growing up', his illness, hospitalisation, rehabilitation at Tadworth, return home and return to school. The early sections on his family and childhood would enable Theo to develop positive stories of identity (Morgan, 2000) and provide a 'safe place to stand' at a distance to trauma (White, 2005). The later sections gave limited but accurate information of his illness and hospitalisation that Grace knew Theo could tolerate. We planned to our roles within the therapy. Grace would regulate Theo's emotions and facilitate his communication. She was a secure attachment figure, and he habitually looked to her to interpret his behavioural signals, gain reassurance or share his joys. I would provide a structure, which gave Theo choice, control and safety in which to explore his situation.

It was particularly important to explore Grace's expectations over the pace and outcome of the therapy. To empower Theo, we would need to invest time in developing his positive stories and allow him to determine the limits of what he wanted to learn about his situation. This placed uncertainty over Grace's GAS goal to increase Theo's knowledge about his situation. We identified this as a potential source of adult frustration and discussed how to protect the therapy process from this and how to continue progress towards this goal after Theo's discharge. We discussed the practicalities of how to facilitate Theo's engagement or withdrawal from activities and topics. We placed a colour-coded 'contents' page in his document to help him guide us. His speech therapist added 'stop'/'keep going' and a 'how I am feeling' tool to his communication aid.

Together, we took great care to ensure that Theo was led by his own needs when working on his autobiography and not by our agenda. The physical set up and social context never assumed that he would choose to work on his autobiography, and it never elevated the status of this work. His autobiography was laid out alongside two of his favourite games. All were equally accessible, and we were equally content to partner him in a game or in working on his book. He was never directed towards his autobiography but was invited to scan and freely choose his activity, and to change his choice at any time. In all but one session, Theo spent most of the time working on his autobiography. Occasionally, he finished with a game.

The intervention involved eight shared sessions with Grace and Theo over four weeks, each lasting 30 to 40 minutes. I also met with Grace alone on five occasions to create the document, to plan, review and evaluate the therapy, and to reflect on her experience of it. Within the shared sessions Theo used a mixture of gesture, expression, vocalisation and his communicator to show us which pages to look at and read to him. Grace and I carefully observed Theo's non-verbal responses to pinpoint areas of importance, curiosity or concern for him. He returned with pleasure to certain areas of text, and we interpreted this as potential positive stories in need of thickening. We offered Theo choices based upon our joint knowledge of him to gain more detail or identify areas of concern. Theo gave explicit consent before any new medical information was offered. After each session, I updated his autobiography with the key ideas that were most meaningful to him. In this way, Theo took control over developing the contents of his autobiography.

Theo developed three significant positive stories (PS) of identity which weaved through the chapters of his document. These positive stories are described in Table 6.1.

Table 6.1 Positive story themes in Theo's document

Positive story 1 (PS1)	His importance to his family, their continual presence through the toughest times in hospital
Positive story 2 (PS2)	His continual role as older brother in caring for his siblings and his cats
Positive story 3 (PS3)	His healing body, the determination of his brain and body to recover from illness and regain physical skills

Theo often used his PS as a way to visit more difficult topics, such as his illness and future schooling. Table 6.2 summarises my sessions with Grace and Theo.

Grace rated her two GAS goals as 'achieved'. Theo had learnt more of his illness, situation and discharge home, and he had a means by which to initiate and control communication over these issues.

Using a 10-point Likert scale (0 = 'none', 10 = 'full'), Grace indicted the degree to which Theo's understanding and their communication over his situation had changed. Her comments show how the autobiography set a context for their communication over his situation. Her ratings are given in Table 6.3.

Table 6.2 Summary of therapy sessions with Grace and Theo

Session 1	This session aimed to determine Theo's engagement with the initial autobiography and to show him he had control over the session activity (autobiography vs. game). Theo readily approached the autobiography and invited us to read it with him. He reviewed the entire contents in sequence. He started to develop PS1 (family support in hospital). He looked at his nasogastric (NG) tube in one photo and gestured to indicate his memory of sensory discomfort. He agreed for me to add his information to his autobiography. Theo then chose a game, perhaps to check these were truly on offer.
Session 2	Theo showed enjoyment of holding and reviewing his autobiography. He added detail to PS1 (family support in hospital). He started PS2 (role as older brother) and considered how this continued through his rehabilitation. Through considering PS1 he reviewed his time in the acute hospital. He did not wish for more information on encephalitis.
Session 3	Theo attended to his autobiography for 40 minutes, starting at the safety of life before his illness. He added detail to PS2 (role as older brother) and PS1 (family support in hospital) as he moved through his autobiography. Whilst considering PS1, he indicated his poor knowledge and recall of his illness and consented to hear a short explanation. Theo pointed and gestured to show his recollection of having his NG tube. Guided by Theo's signs of engagement, we focussed on his memories about having his tube and its removal. This introduced a new positive story 3 (PS3) about the determination of his body and brain to recover. Theo remained highly focussed on this new positive story, and we expanded it under his guidance. Within this story, he visited the sections on his rehabilitation and discharge home. He consented for me to add a visual countdown to discharge. He quickly disengaged when we revealed the page about his future school, indicating he did not wish to think about this.
Session 4	Theo reviewed the sections associated with PS1 (family support in hospital) and PS2 (role as older brother). After thinking about these positive stories, he visited the section on his future education, and indicated he was anxious. Together we identified his main questions and he asked Grace to research answers for these. He made a plan to see photographs of potential schools in preference to visiting them in person.
Session 5	Theo reviewed his whole autobiography in sequence. By thinking about PS2 (role as older brother), he visited the topic of his discharge home, particularly his change of bedroom. He rested briefly on the topic of his new school and then indicated he felt too anxious to think about this today.

Session 6	Theo reviewed the section of his stay in the acute hospital. Whilst thinking about PS3 (brain and body recovery), Theo asked Grace to describe her memories of this period. Theo traced the recovery of his skills through his rehabilitation. He then chose to hear a little about meningoencephalitis.
Session 7	Theo was keen to come to his session. Grace reported he had been visibly low in mood and less motivated in his rehabilitation that morning. Theo directed his autobiography to review the acute stages of his encephalitis. He then disengaged, indicating a need to use the toilet. Within this privacy with Grace, he became tearful. He chose to return and engaged in sensory play. After a while, he tolerated my closed questions to identify the following concerns: • I want to know more about encephalitis. • Do I still have encephalitis? • I want to know more about my brain learning new skills Under his direction, Grace and I answered these concerns. Theo indicated that he wanted to ask a medical professional, and we made a plan for this. Theo looked visibly tired but relieved. As I waved goodbye, he reapproached me, carefully interlocked his fingers with mine, made eye contact and smiled. Grace and I interpreted that he had greatly valued the session and the plan we had created.
	At this stage, Grace and I identified the information to offer Theo about his encephalitis. This was offered to him by a specialist brain injury nurse and written up to be offered for his autobiography.
Session 8	The last therapeutic session, held two days before Theo's discharge. Theo reviewed the topic of his discharge. We extended PS3 (his brain's recovery of skills) through the later stages of his rehabilitation, adding the photos of horse riding he had brought to evidence this. We extended this positive story into his future life at home. He did not wish to review the additional information on encephalitis. Instead, he chose to add it at the back of his autobiography in a separate section. I collated Theo's feedback on the therapy. Theo indicated he planned to take his autobiography home. We reviewed where he would keep it and with whom he would share it.

Table 6.3 Grace's ratings of therapy outcome using Likert scale

Item to Be Rated	*Rating Taken Prior to Start of Psychotherapy*	*Rating Taken at Completion of Psychotherapy*
Theo's overall understanding of what has happened and his current situation	3–4	8–9
Your awareness of how much he understands of what has happened and his current situation	5–6	7
How much he can initiate and control communication over his situation	1–2	10, "with autobiography in quiet setting"
How much he can indicate what he does/does not want to know about his situation	1–2	9–10 "with his autobiography It's great he can skip sections"

Table 6.4 Theo's ratings of therapy outcome

Question	*Like*	*Not Sure*	*Not Like*
How do you feel about your book?	X		
How do you feel about the section on 'You'?	X		
How do you feel about the section on 'My Illness'?		X	
How do you feel about the section on 'My Stay in Hospital'?		X	
How do you feel about the section on 'My Stay at Tadworth'?	X		
How do you feel about the section on 'Going Home'?		X	
How do you feel about the section on 'Going to School'?	X		
How do you feel about these sessions to look at your book?	X		
Do you want to take the book home?	Yes		
Do you want other people to look at the book with you when you get home?	Mum Dad Bubba Grandpa	Daniel Emily	

Theo gave his feedback by choosing one of three responses (like/not sure/do not like) to a series of questions. This is given in Table 6.4.

Reflections

Theo's feedback shows his ambivalence towards the difficult content of his journey. It also shows he felt attached to his autobiographical document, despite its challenging contents. I believe Theo's high degree of control in accessing and developing his autobiography was critical to his attachment. In its final form, the autobiography told his story of the resources he used to survive his illness and brain injury. Within its pages, Theo presents positive and authentic self-representations that have endured and adapted through acute adversity. Theo's autobiography symbolises another authentic self-representation of his courage to explore and learn about his situation, as witnessed by Grace.

Theo's dependency on us to build his document raised additional clinical and ethical dilemmas about protecting him from our own therapy goals. SNT always carries a tension between establishing the adult goals to improve the child's understanding and communication, and handing control of therapy outcome to the child. It is critical to manage this tension at all stages of the therapy to establish and maintain the child's control. This minimises the risk of the child feeling influenced by adult expectations to visit distressing information, which would support the dominant narrative of disempowerment and victimisation (White, 2005).

As the therapy progressed, I became uncomfortably aware that I was relying greatly on Grace's resources to protect Theo from her own goals. On reflection, I should have identified more explicitly what to do if adult expectation had crept in to influence the therapy.

As with many therapeutic interventions, SNT carries the risk of the child feeling answerable to the adult expectations of the therapy. In SNT, this risk is minimised by explicitly empowering the child as much as possible, but it cannot be eliminated altogether. This inherent risk within SNT needs to be balanced against the risks of not offering the therapy. SNT allows a child to gain a greater factual understanding of their situation than an orientation script, and it establishes a context for child-centred communication through which to learn more from their family. It also attends to the developmental process behind the child's identity.

Without SNT, a child may only learn about his or her brain injury through adult-led 'brain injury education' or in separate, problem-saturated contexts where his or her needs arise. These routes are an important part of rehabilitation, but they demand more resources from the child than SNT and should be implemented with this in mind.

References

Caplan, B., Bogner, J., Brenner, L., Beadle, E., Ownsworth, T., Fleming, J., & Shum, D. (2016). The impact of traumatic brain injury on self-identity: A systematic review of the evidence for self-concept changes. *Journal of Head Trauma Rehabilitation, 31*(2), E12–E25.

Gan, C., Gargaro, J., Kreutzer, J., Boschen, K., & Wright, F. (2010). Development and preliminary evaluation of a structured family system intervention for adolescents with brain injury and their families. *Brain Injury, 24*(4), 651–663.

Gracey, F., Evans, J., & Malley, D. (2009). Capturing process and outcome in complex rehabilitation interventions: A "Y-shaped" model. *Neuropsychological Rehabilitation, 19*(6), 867–890.

Gracey, F., Longworth, C., & Psaila, K. (2016). A provisional transdiagnostic cognitive behavioural model of post brain injury emotional adjustment. *Neuro-Disability and Psychotherapy, 3*(2), 154–185.

Harter, S. (2012). *The construction of the self: Developmental and sociocultural foundations*. New York: Guilford Press.

Krasny-Pacini, A., Limond, J., Evans, J., Hiebel, J., Bendjelida, K., & Chevignard, M. (2015). Self-awareness assessment during cognitive rehabilitation in children with acquired brain injury: A feasibility study and proposed model of child anosognosia. *Disability and Rehabilitation, 37*(22), 2092–2106.

Limond, J., Adlam, A., & Cormack, M. (2014). A model for pediatric neurocognitive interventions: Considering the role of development and maturation in rehabilitation planning. *The Clinical Neuropsychologist, 28*(2), 181–198.

Lloyd, O., Ownsworth, T., Fleming, J., & Zimmer-Gembeck, M. (2015). Awareness deficits in children and adolescents after traumatic brain injury: A systematic review. *The Journal of Head Trauma Rehabilitation, 30*(5), 311–323.

Morgan, A. (2000). *What is narrative therapy*. Adelaide: Dulwich Centre Publications.

Ownsworth, T., & Clare, L. (2006). The association between awareness deficits and rehabilitation outcome following acquired brain injury. *Clinical Psychology Review*, *26*(6), 783–795.

Perkins, A. (2015). Psychological support using narrative psychotherapy for children with brain injury. In J. Reed, K. Byard, & H. Fine (Eds.), *Neuropsychological rehabilitation of childhood brain injury: A practical guide* (pp. 215–236). New York: Springer.

Wade, S., & Hung, A. (2015). Online family problem solving for adolescent traumatic brain injury. In J. Reed, K. Byard, & H. Fine (Eds.), *Neuropsychological rehabilitation of childhood brain injury: A practical guide* (pp. 43–59). New York: Springer.

Waldron, B., Casserly, L., & O'Sullivan, C. (2013). Cognitive behavioural therapy for depression and anxiety in adults with acquired brain injury. What works for whom? *Neuropsychological Rehabilitation*, *23*(1), 64–101.

Walsh, F. (2012). Family resilience: Strengths forged through adversity. In F. Walsh (Ed.), *Normal family processes: Growing diversity and complexity* (pp. 399–427). New York: Guilford Press.

White, M. (2005). Children, trauma and subordinate story line development. *International Journal of Narrative Therapy & Community Work*, (3–4), 10–21.

Wolfe, K., Bigler, E., Dennis, M., Gerhardt, C., Rubin, K., Taylor, H. G., . . . Yeates, K. (2014). Self-awareness of peer-rated social attributes in children with traumatic brain injury. *Journal of Pediatric Psychology*, *40*(3), 272–284.

Yeates, G., Henwood, K., Gracey, F., & Evans, J. (2007). Awareness of disability after acquired brain injury and the family context. *Neuropsychological Rehabilitation*, *17*(2), 151–173.

Chapter 7

Mindfulness interventions for people with aphasia – case evidence from individual and group therapy formats

Maristella Crielesi[1], Lauren Roche, Giulia Monopoli, Giles N. Yeates, Stefano Monte

Introduction

Meeting the person with aphasia: rehabilitation and psychotherapy

Aphasia is the partial or complete loss of language skills in its production and/or comprehension processes, resulting from an acquired brain injury or degenerative condition. When a person is confronted by the challenges of aphasia, their quality of life can be undermined through simultaneous neurological, psychological and psycho-social difficulties. Aphasia risks reducing the influence which a person can exercise on what was once a two-way interaction. In the eyes of others, it is probable that people with aphasia will be found to be of unsound mind, instead of being perceived as interlocutors with expressive abilities and a brain which still thinks.

Communication can be understood as a "joint activity of actor and partner, who consciously and intentionally cooperate to build together the meaning of their interaction". The agents of the interaction are together and to the same extent actively engaged in the construction of a shared meaning. What happens when a person totally or partially loses the possibility of being considered by the other as an active subject in the linguistic communicative interaction? Which consequences does the compromising of the linguistic activity involve in the other aspects of life?

Even after the conclusion of functional rehabilitation programs, these people may find themselves faced with a radical change in their identity, which seems to promise limited future expectations in the social and physical activities, as a consequence established by the disability.

The characteristics of aphasia are also unique when compared with other forms of impairment and disability. It is hardly recognizable and very different both from person to person and from moment to moment, even in the same person because it depends on the levels of stress and fatigue. Persons with aphasia who do not report visible physical damages seem to find themselves at a crossroads in different public situations. The choice of a person with aphasia is between withdrawing from relationships "because aphasia is a difficult problem to explain" or risking and exposing himself, often perceiving his condition as a fault: "Excuse me, but I am aphasic".

Mindfulness and aphasia

Mindfulness has been defined by Bishop. The first component identified by the authors is the self-regulation of attention, in order to maintain it in the immediate experience, allowing a better possibility of recognizing mental events in the present moment. The second component described consists in adopting a new orientation, which makes the patient reconsider his own experience of the present, characterized by three elements: curiosity, openness and acceptance.

Starting from this definition, it is possible to assert that the potential contribution provided by the integrated mindfulness-based approach to people with aphasia is to make direct contact with their experiences, even if they are unpleasant and tiring, without the need to reject them. The ability to pay attention in a conscious way in the present moment is trained, exhorting the abstinence from judgements.

It becomes clear that, in this reflective modality, the contents which emerge to the mind are not the totality of the inner self. This aspect, combined with the awareness that what we think is produced by our mental activity, and may therefore not correspond to reality, makes the disidentification from the contents generated by the mind possible. The distance of the patient from his own mental contents allows the creation of space, so that the suspension of normal reaction patterns and judgements, sources of profound suffering, can take place. Only by understanding the functioning of our mind and by having the possibility, offered by the mode of being, to look at our mental activity as something which does not coincide with ourselves, do we lay the foundations for our freedom. Being able to choose not to be driven by our own thoughts allows us to be disconnected from conditioning and guarantees us the possibility of acting according to a truly personal and free choice.

A small collection of case studies have been published on the application of mindfulness meditation in the context of aphasia. The impact of a mindfulness intervention on divided attention in people with aphasia has been investigated by Orenstein and colleagues (2012), and Laures-Gore and Marshall (2016) reported improvements on both psychophysiological (heart rate, heart-rate variability), cognitive (decreased impulsivity, improved attention) and communication performance (word production, phrase length, word generation) measures in an individual with aphasia (14 years post stroke) following a five-day mindfulness meditation training. This group extended their approach to a small group study, finding a superior but non-significant difference in the five-day mindfulness training group versus controls (Marshall, Laures-Gore, & Love, 2018). In a post-stroke aphasia case study reported by Dickenson and colleagues (2017), significant reductions in anxiety alongside communication gains (improvements in confrontation naming picture description and repetition) were reported. The authors made the case that approaches such as mindfulness meditation may offer a way to break the disabling negative interactions between anxiety and exacerbation of communication restrictions in people with aphasia.

Exploring the contribution of mindfulness interventions for people with aphasia

Mindfulness interventions can be delivered via both individual sessions and group formats, and both approaches feature in the studies reported earlier. In this paper, we explore in detail the contributions of both intervention formats in supporting the psychological needs of people with aphasia. To this end, we present a detailed descriptive case study (clinical work undertaken by Lauren Roche), followed by a case series analysis of five participants in a mindfulness group intervention conducted by Maristella Crielesi and Giulia Monopoli.

Illustrative case study

Case introduction: Rose (a pseudonym), a 67-year-old white British woman residing in an older-adult care home, was referred to the local neuropsychology service by a speech and language therapist (SaLT) who was concerned about her withdrawal from therapy, increasing distress and declining mood. In the care home, Rose was receiving input from a community rehabilitation team, including a physiotherapist (PT), an occupational therapist (OT) and a speech and language therapist (SaLT). Rose was additionally assessed and treated by a trainee clinical psychologist under the supervision of a consultant neuropsychologist.

Presenting complaints: Rose suffered a left middle cerebral artery infarct in June 2014 and consequently experienced expressive aphasia and significant right-sided weakness. She was referred to neuropsychology services following observations of increasing frustration and distress in formal speech and language therapy sessions, as well as observations of withdrawal and variable mood within the home.

History: Rose had no known previous mental health history and few physical health concerns before her stroke. She smoked but had stopped doing so since her admission. She had been retired and lived independently, having lost her husband two years previously; they had one son, now an adult, who lived locally and remained in frequent contact.

Assessment: Expressive aphasia was evident, and other neuropsychological difficulties were hypothesized, but it was decided with Rose that formal neuropsychological testing would not be a priority, because attempts at formal speech and language assessment during her acute rehabilitation had been discontinued as Rose had found it highly distressing. She continued to find focused therapy sessions difficult and so it seemed likely that further testing would also be distressing.

Furthermore, it is likely that any information about her optimal cognitive functioning would be invalidated by such a high emotive factor in her presentation. Assessment therefore consisted of multi-source data collection, including review of SaLT notes, observations and discussions with Rose, the care staff and her son.

Discussions with Rose: At times Rose was able to form complete coherent sentences, but she also frequently struggled to express herself beyond single words, or noises. At these times, frustration was evident and she frequently repeated the phrase "I don't know, I don't know". It took several prompts at this stage to re-engage her in other topics of conversation. Her understanding of others' speech appeared to be good; although her frustration was evident at times, she followed conversation, responded appropriately and was evidently engaged. Rose could recall activities she enjoyed but struggled to generate ideas of new activities and returned repeatedly to unrealistic past activities. She was also able to communicate that her mood fluctuates: sometimes she has good thoughts and sometimes 'bad' ones such as "I don't want to be here", of equal frequency. She noted that her self-esteem was low.

Rose described herself previously as a quiet, private woman who was easy-going, habitual and family-oriented and who enjoyed keeping house. Her son agreed with this description, adding that she was a perfectionist with high self-standards.

Speech and language therapy observations: Comments throughout these notes indicated that Rose was struggling to adjust to her post-stroke experience: she described feeling that her recovery had plateaued, yet was finding it hard to come to terms with the disability she was left with and the long-term change in status. She wished her son and brother not to see her because 'she was not herself'; she was embarrassed at others seeing her like this, both friends/family and new people, which meant she was reluctant to leave her room or to have visitors. She described a range of emotions – anger, anxiety, worry – but 'didn't know what to do with them'. She was 'tired of trying'.

These session notes also indicated the issues within therapy sessions – the last few sessions had been ended prematurely because of "fixation on errors and mistakes to the point where she is unable to move beyond this and the task needs to be abandoned". The time of engagement per session was decreasing.

Case conceptualization: The boxes on the left in Figure 7.1 were clinical hypotheses developed by the SaLT and the author as to Rose's current difficulties that could further explain her own explanations, which are documented in the boxes in bold on the right.

In consideration of the literature outlined earlier, ruminative practices were observable as Rose switched between thoughts about her past, and what she had been able to achieve in contrast to now, and her future, towards which she felt hopeless ("I don't know what to do"). These thoughts were also laden with evaluative judgements such as "I *should* be able to complete this task" and fusion with emotive content: "I cannot bear for people to see me like this". Rose's repetition of "I don't know what I'm going to do" also seemed to summarize her low

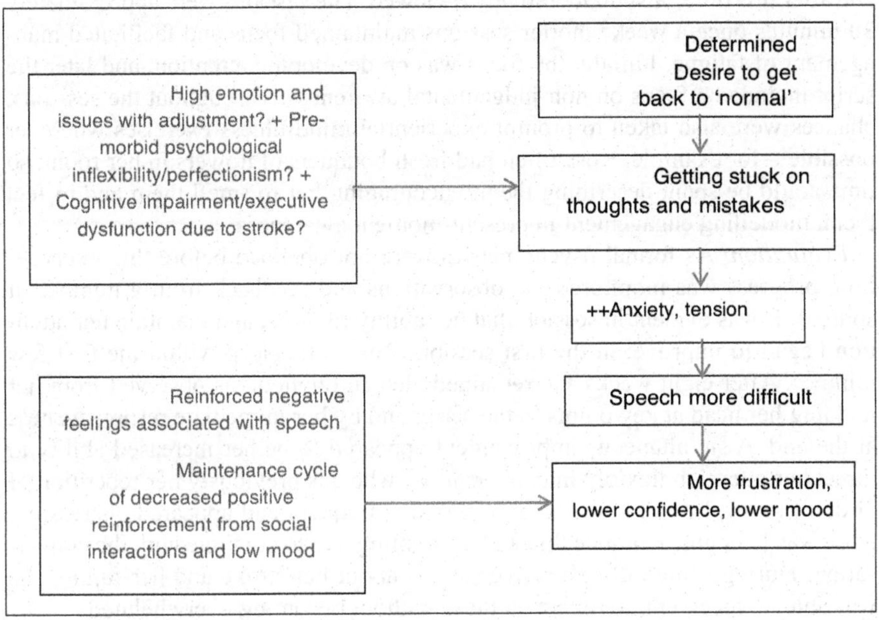

Figure 7.1 Detailed case study formulation

sense of control and self-esteem. Rose displayed attachment to functional outcomes particularly in her therapy sessions, which led to significant distress when these could not be achieved; this process seemed to be exacerbated by decreased emotional regulation and reduced ability to flexibly direct her attention. Furthermore, this intense focus was limiting her ability to contact other experiences in the present. Rose was relying on habitual coping behaviours (problem/task focused) despite these being less effective in such a different context. We considered that her withdrawal was an understandable but ultimately unhelpful attempt to avoid the uncomfortable aspects of her experience, but which also resulted in reduced positive reinforcement and a limited behavioural repertoire. We also noted that these processes were likely further exacerbated by the formal, functional rehabilitation approach employed at the time.

Intervention: Given the formulation of her current experiences as outlined earlier, it was considered that mindfulness could be a pragmatic way of working with Rose given her expressive aphasia as well as a positive approach, with no noted harmful effects in the literature, and diverse beneficial effects that could potentially help with functional rehabilitation as well as alternative outcomes such as improved personal wellbeing and decreased distress.

Rose completed eight sessions of mindfulness practice, in which the author read a mindfulness script out loud. During this time, speech therapy was suspended, and after this time, we collaboratively reviewed. The sessions were approximately 30 minutes once a week; shorter sessions maintained focus and facilitated management of fatigue. Initially the focus was on developing attention, and later the script included a focus on non-judgemental awareness. Throughout the sessions, chances were also taken to prompt experiential mindfulness exercises wherever possible – for example, Rose often had fresh bouquets of flowers in her room, so time could be spent describing them, encouraging her to smell them and to feel them, modelling engagement in present-moment awareness.

Evaluation: As formal psychometrics were not obtained before this intervention, progress was monitored via observations and feedback from a number of sources. It was evident in session that her ability to direct and maintain her attention began to improve: in the first session, Rose fell asleep within the first few minutes. After eight weeks she remained alert throughout, as observed from her nodding her head at key points in the script and by her immediate responsiveness at the end. A simultaneous improvement appeared to be her increased ability to direct her attention flexibly in conversation: whereas previously her repetition of "I don't know, I don't know what to do" was frequent and appeared distressing, Rose was later able to notice this with prompting and to continue with the conversation. During some difficult conversations about her stroke and her future, she was able, to an extent, to reflect on these without becoming overwhelmed.

Rose herself reported some change at the end of the eight weeks – she noted that her mood was still very variable but that she had more good times than bad. She also reported that her self-esteem was mostly good, in contrast to low self-esteem noted at the beginning. Rose described the mindfulness practice as 'slow, slow slow' in contrast to her normal mind full of thoughts.

Her son kept in regular email contact and noted that "Generally (her) mood has been a little better . . . a little less frustration". Similarly, he noted that "(she) is still making steady progress with speech which is great, and is perhaps learning not to give up quite so readily" – this despite the discontinuation of formal speech therapy. These observations were in line with the aims of the intervention. Although there are obvious queries about demand characteristics and desirability bias, at no stage was her son asked for specific reports on these topics.

The care home continued to note fluctuating mood with limited willingness to engage in group activities. A joint evaluative session with speech and language therapy took place after the eight-week intervention. It was noted that Rose was bright in mood, and her motivation to engage again in speech therapy was increased. However, her cognitive impairments remained obvious: a trial using an iPad to communicate was not successful as she was not able to retain her train of thought and type her communications effectively, becoming perseverative about particular letters or words. She did not appear as fixed on her mistakes and her stroke as in previous SaLT sessions, but she did become progressively more frustrated: it became clear that even though her mood and her relationship with her thoughts seemed to have improved, her ability to engage in further speech therapy remained impaired. This final collaborative session led to a decision to refocus the ongoing interventions to emphasize wellbeing rather than functional ability. Formal speech therapy was therefore stopped.

The reformulated, client-centred goals were shared with and supported by other members of the team, including the OT and the care home staff. A key worker was assigned to Rose, who agreed to be briefed in and to maintain mindfulness practice via a number of scripts and a CD left for Rose. Her son engaged in a discussion about the use of mindfulness applications on his iPad which he already used on some of his visits with her. The home also agreed to find a 'befriender' for Rose, to encourage social interaction and to facilitate informal practice of her speech. The Activities Lead timetabled in some 1:1 time to spend with Rose on pleasant tasks such as self-care activities and independent living tasks, with a view to encourage present-moment awareness and increase her sense of control.

Follow-up: Observations during a visit three weeks' post intervention indicated maintained attentional gains during a mindfulness practice, objectively bright mood and subjective acknowledgement that mood was variable still but mostly good. Staff reported that she had been out of the home on a group trip and another was planned, which was considerable given her previous distress at such suggestions: although not able to correlate this specifically with the intervention, this is nonetheless anecdotal evidence in line with the hypothesis that willingness to accept her experience, increased ability to regulate emotions and choose valued behaviours would be a positive and iterative process; it is hoped that further desensitization to negative affect and increased positive affect should continue to facilitate her engagement and improve her quality of life.

Mindfulness group evaluation

Service context: The Create Integration Resiliency Possibility (CIRP) – Aphasia Center of Turin pursues the central objective of improving participation in the life of the person, in line with Life Participation Approach to Aphasia (LPAA, Kagan, ref). Survivors are invited to collaborate actively in all phases of the intervention, starting from the identification of the objectives through an analysis of the demand, and to commit to their realization together with the operators.

The center, which deals mainly with cases of aphasia caused by stroke, works according to the bio-psycho-social perspective, which is able to look beyond the cognitive aspects of aphasia, in order to conceive the change also in psychological, relational and social terms. According to this perspective, the consequences of aphasia determine a change on the whole personal and social sphere, which makes it necessary to facilitate a learning process on the new condition, in order to be able to integrate the limits with the residual capacities. This learning often does not happen spontaneously, but rather requires a 'transformation', possibly thanks to the psychotherapeutic tool.

As in any clinical environment, even in cases of stroke and aphasia, it is necessary to explore which interventions, and which modalities, can be proposed to achieve the best level of wellbeing in everyday life.

Some of the outcomes of stroke and aphasia involve changes, including lifestyle habits, the role in the family and the experience which the patient has with himself. A survivor's realization that some of these physical and linguistic changes are stable and profoundly enduring often generates suffering.

One of the objectives which seems to be shared at this level, when the individual is confronted with the impossibility of 'returning exactly as before', is to improve the relationship which the person has with his own experience of disability. In this way, it is possible to lay the foundations to facilitate the recognition of the person's own potentialities, beyond the limits set by aphasia.

A practice which can be useful to improve the relationship with the experience of the person, even if it is unpleasant or painful, is the *mindfulness* practice.

This paper is the first exploration of a group intervention, based on mindfulness in the CIRP. The clinical work reported here is influenced by a previous Canadian study. The main aim of this study is to investigate the impact of a mindfulness-based group on the psychological functioning in four stroke survivors with aphasia.

Service context: This study was initiated to investigate the efficacy of an intervention based on mindfulness applied in the context of aphasia. Starting from January 2011, clinical practices based on mindfulness were introduced within the activities of the center. It was initially provided individual psychotherapy sessions, in which one of the tools used was mindfulness, to promote integration among bodily sensations, emotions and thoughts, cultivating a mode of moment-by-moment awareness. Starting from the direct experience of these moments as described in a Canadian evaluation of a mindfulness group for patients who had suffered a stroke (Moustgaard et al., 2007), an intervention was designed and built for patients with moderate linguistic deficits. In cases of mild aphasia, the linguistic deficits do not seem to apparently result in a significant change for the identity of the person, who returns, to the extent which it is possible, to the working and social life preceding the traumatic event. However, the team has frequently found that the quality of life subjectively perceived by the person with aphasia can bring out aspects of a more silent and less obvious discomfort, compared with what those around them can read and see, especially in cases in which the deficit is less severe. The weight of this condition can emerge from comparison with the past and the difficulty in accepting the limits imposed by aphasia. Besides these aspects, the mild linguistic deficit presents a new facet: it can be almost invisible on an objective level even in the closest people; the lack of recognition by others of the consequences of a deficit which "is perceived only in some cases" can increase tensions, worries, anxiety and a sense of inadequacy.

The mindfulness group is born, starting from the need to offer the patient new ways to relate to his own experience after stroke and aphasia, and its purpose is the recognition and acceptance by patients of their limits, together with the identification of their resources in the new situation.

Mindfulness group for people with aphasia: In line with the content of the LPAA principles, the general objective of the intervention focuses on the dimension of interpersonal relationships and social participation. The main purpose of the research is to identify the effectiveness of a mindfulness-based program with a group of aphasic patients after a stroke. The achievement of "awareness in the new condition of life" is considered the key to lead to the possible resolution of the internal conflict which breaks out when expectations about life do not correspond to how life is in reality. The intent is not to 'get rid of' something, but to experience 'being in the present moment' in a climate of openness and acceptance, without the need to be anchored to judgements. From this way of being reflective, a fundamental process emerges, and it becomes possible to be aware of the fact that the activities of our mind are not the totality of what we are.

The specific objectives of the intervention are three: to experiment with a different relationship with one's own experience, allowing it to be what it is, without judging it and without having to modify it; to develop a greater sensitivity for the recognition of one's emotions and achieve a greater balance in their management; and to foster better access to possible inner resources and personal qualities through a greater ability to get in touch with oneself on an emotional, sensory and mental level.

The chosen setting is that of the group, in order to provide an intermediate social network able to unite a more clinical/rehabilitative environment to a more personal one. The group also represents the opportunity to share psychological and communicative aspects in a context of exchange in which active participation is envisaged.

Given the target to which it is addressed, it was also chosen to use the small group to facilitate a simple and effective communication between the members during the meetings.

Before embarking on the group process, participants were offered an individual phase of preparation for the proposed intervention, in which personal goals, motivation, expectations and fears were discussed and shared.

The Mindfulness-Based Therapy intervention of the mindfulness group was structured starting from the contents of the Mindfulness-Based Cognitive Therapy (MBCT) previously introduced. The topics envisaged by the MBCT protocol were followed; nevertheless, given the important differences compared with the target for which it was built, variations were made, so that the protocol could better respond to the needs of the patients with aphasia to whom it was applied. Taking into account the communicative difficulties of the participants, the use of the SCA techniques (Supported Conversation for Adults with Aphasia) was foreseen by the group leader. They are proposed in order to create an accessible communicative environment for a better chance of relating to the person with aphasia and are explicitly designed for people who 'know more than they can say', in order to allow them the expression of opinions and emotions, using and revealing the communication skills still available. In addition, all the paper material provided to the participants was made as suitable as possible for people with linguistic deficits, using a simple language and a writing font size appropriate for easier reading and understanding.

The sessions included different forms of meditation which alternated with moments of reflection starting from the experiences of the participants; psycho-education moments dedicated to aphasia and stroke have also been included. Investigating the possibilities of movement of the participants after the stroke, it was chosen to exclude yoga exercises from the program. The meditation exercises, excluding the walking meditation, were all performed in a sitting position because not all the participants could access the lying position without consequences.

Participants: The target recipients of the research-intervention were people who became aphasic after a stroke, selected among the users of the center who met the criteria for inclusion in the project.

The criteria for group inclusion established that the time since the stroke occurred was at least six months and that the consequent aphasia was of homogeneous production. Those with conscience disorders or other neurological disorders (such as dementia) and those with impaired language comprehension skills were excluded. A group consisting of four patients meeting the criteria and motivated to take part and to contribute to the analysis of the efficacy of the proposed treatment was therefore established. Three of the participants were on their first intervention at the facility. One of them (G.M.) had previously been followed by the center for some psychological counseling sessions. For the duration of the treatment, the group did not take part in other psychotherapeutic pathways or interventions.

The group comprised two men and two women aged between 47 and 78 with a medium-light production deficit (Table 7.1). Understanding is generally preserved, even if, at times, it is necessary to reiterate the communicative message. The four people have different reading and writing problems; for one of the subjects the writing skill is very compromised. None of the participants had motor outcomes which led to the use of wheelchairs or other walking aids; however, the movement of the right side of the body was still difficult as regards the performance of certain activities.

Procedure: The research is open to monitoring the potentials and limitations of an intervention such as mindfulness in the context of aphasia. Mindfulness is

Table 7.1 Description of the participants

	M.B.	*A.F.*	*C.F.*	*G.M.*
Age	47	69	59	78
Gender	Female	Male	Male	Female
Time since stroke	17 months	13 months	12 months	27 months
Type of aphasia	Production	Production	Production	Production
Schooling	15	11	4	n.d.
Caregiver	Nobody	Wife	Wife	Friend (woman)

therefore introduced into the group and used as a specific active element of which consequences and effects can be detected. This is a pre-experiment, as it makes use of a single group of participants and two evaluation tests, a pre-treatment and a post-treatment one. The research-intervention approach was used with the aim of studying the therapeutic process on the one hand and evaluating its effectiveness on the other, using evaluation tools repeated over time (T0, start of intervention; T1, end of intervention).

Before the beginning of the intervention, all relevant informed consent forms were gathered for the participation in the clinical research-intervention and for the treatment of personal data. The people involved were aware of the aims of the research and their personal contribution in taking part in it. They were informed about the full freedom to withdraw from the project at any time they deemed it necessary.

The mindfulness group provided group meetings, lasting two hours each, once a week for eight weeks. At the meetings there were the four participants and the psychologist, psychotherapist and mindfulness teacher.

As users of the Aphasia Center, the people who took part in the mindfulness group had received the prescribed test for taking charge at a pre-treatment stage. Once assigned to the group treatment based on mindfulness, in an initial individual phase, the participants were informed of the terms of the intervention and were introduced in advance to the mindfulness approach. Because the meetings were videotaped, all the participants filled out the form for the release of the scheduled video and audio recordings. During these individual meetings, specific tests for the mindfulness group project were administered to each participant, in order to obtain the pre-treatment data for the research.

In each of the eight meetings, a specific theme was addressed: the planned activities alternated between moments of sharing and reflection and moments dedicated to the mindfulness meditation. At the end of the sessions, the participants received material summarizing the contents and the topics addressed. In addition, some meditation exercises were given to do at home during the week (with the help of CDs provided at the meetings), along with the compilation of some diary forms, according to the communication abilities of the participants. Four weeks after the end of the treatment, a further debriefing group meeting was scheduled in which the initial individual objectives, shared during the first session, were recalled and a group discussion on the mindfulness group experience was made possible.

This phase was followed by the re-test phase, in which all the tests used for the assessment phase were administered for a second time, both those specific to the Aphasia Center and those directly related to the research-intervention.

Measures: The main purpose of the evaluation was to observe any changes in terms of perceived psychological wellbeing and to identify possible variations in attention-related cognitive functions. To do this, a series of specific tests for the detection of the emotional state and some tests on attention were used.

The tests selected and used provide the following information:

- Mood state by direct administration BDI-II (Beck Depression Inventory Revised; and VAMS (Visual Analog Mood Scale);
- Mood status by indirect administration (SADQ-10 Stroke Aphasia Depression Questionnaire 10 items);
- State anxiety and trait anxiety (STAIX – State-Trait Anxiety Inventory);
- Quality of life (SS-QoL – Stroke Specific Quality of Life Scale);
- Mindfulness skills in its five components (FFMQ – Five Facet Mindfulness Questionnaire);
- Visual and spatial search capacity and attention capacities TMT (Trail Making Test) and TMA (Test of Attention Matrices,)

Preliminary results: The preliminary research data of each person are presented here, with more detailed subsequent analyses to be shared in a future paper. The overall scores for participants on all measures pre- and post-intervention are shown in Tables 7.2 through 7.4.

Global scores obtained in performed tests are described in more detail in Tables 7.2, 7.3 and 7.4.

Table 7.2 Depression and anxiety detection: results in the T0 and T1 phases for each participant

	M.B.		*A.F.*		*C.F.*		*G.M.*	
	T0	*T1*	*T0*	*T1*	*T0*	*T1*	*T0*	*T1*
BDI-II	12	10	7	6	9	7	7	10
SADQ-10	n.d.	n.d.	14	8	19	16	7	4
STAI X-1	48	34	32	26	33	20	35	31
STAI X-2	55	53	36	30	32	25	44	41

Table 7.3 Mindfulness and quality of life: scores for each participant in the T0 and T1 phases

	M.B.		*A.F.*		*C.F.*		*M.G.*	
	T0	*T1*	*T0*	*T1*	*T0*	*T1*	*T0*	*T1*
FFMQ: Obs	28	34	34	36	12	22	25	20
FFMQ: Des	34	40	29	25	28	34	31	29
FFMQ: AC	25	23	20	25	25	36	31	29
FFMQ: NJ	24	25	25	31	34	40	32	27
FFMQ: NR	17	15	28	26	31	34	25	34
FFMQ: Total	128	137	136	143	130	166	144	139

	M.B.		A.F.		C.F.		M.G.	
	T0	T1	T0	T1	T0	T1	T0	T1
SSQoL: En	13	13	10	12	14	15	3	10
SSQoL: FR	7	13	13	14	15	13	8	6
SSQoL: Comm	18	22	13	19	19	22	11	14
SSQoL: Mov	30	29	28	30	30	30	30	28
SSQoL: Mo	18	16	24	25	18	25	16	20
SSQoL: Per	5	14	15	14	13	11	12	12
SSQoL: PC	25	25	25	25	25	25	2	25
SSQoL: SR	23	25	19	20	24	25	13	16
SSQoL: Tho	6	13	6	9	9	13	7	11
SSQoL: UA	20	25	25	25	23	25	20	25
SSQoL: Sig	15	15	14	15	15	15	15	15
SSQoL: J	15	15	12	13	14	13	13	15
SSQoL: Total	195	225	204	221	219	232	153	197

Note: FFMQ (Five Facet Mindfulness Questionnaire): Obs = Observe, Des = Describe, AC = Act Consciously, NJ = No Judgement, NR = No Reaction; SS-QOL (Stroke Specific Quality of Life Scale): En = Energy, FR = Familiar Role, Comm = Communication, Mov = Movement, Mo = Mood, Per = Personality, PC = Personal Care, SR = Social Role, Tho = Thought, AS = Upper Arts, Sig = Sight, J = Job.

Table 7.4 Results Attention skills

	M.B.		A.F.		C.F.		G.M.	
	T0	T1	T0	T1	T0	T1	T0	T1
Attention matrices	41	46	47	47	31	39	19	24
TMT Test 1	65	52	56	40	120	86	180	185
TMT Alternate	118	40	111	69	285	184	600	280

Note: Scores in the attention matrices and the time taken for the two tests of the Trail Making Test (TMT) (measured in seconds) for each participant in the T0 and T1 times

In the following subparagraphs, some aspects of each participant are presented: a brief description of life and situation, aphasia experience and individual objectives and results. Graphs aim to suggest the occurred change following mindfulness-based treatment. The scores obtained in the various tests administered are described in more detail in Tables 7.2, 7.3 and 7.4.

Case M.B.: MB was a 47-year-old woman who had two hemorrhagic strokes following hysterectomy surgery. She had mild expressive aphasia, but her comprehension of language was very high. She lived alone; after stroke she moved her home near her mother's home. She was the founder and manager of a private residence for people with mental illness. She had recovered her autonomy, but she no longer felt the same as she used to be. She was struggling in her work; the requests were the same as before but she thought that her resources were no longer the same. She had little social life. She preferred quiet places; noise and confusion limited her communication possibilities. M.B.'s goals were:

- To increase the ability to manage difficult situations in life, stress, conflicts and ordinary and extraordinary problems.
- To be able to stay in the present moment, without comparing with the past.
- To have a different relation with her current experience.

After the end of the group, in the individual meeting, M.B. described the experience as having been positive. She found important psychological and communicative aspects in the group.

M.B. recognized her ability to be in the present and to handle difficult situations, especially on an emotional level.

Difficulties continued in the perception of communication skills, and M.B. felt that her physical energy had not improved. This suggested that the third goal was not achieved.

The achieved subjective goals seemed to be in line with some of the proposed results. Reference was made in particular to the reduction of anxiety, especially anxiety of state, and to the increase in mindfulness ability. Being able to observe

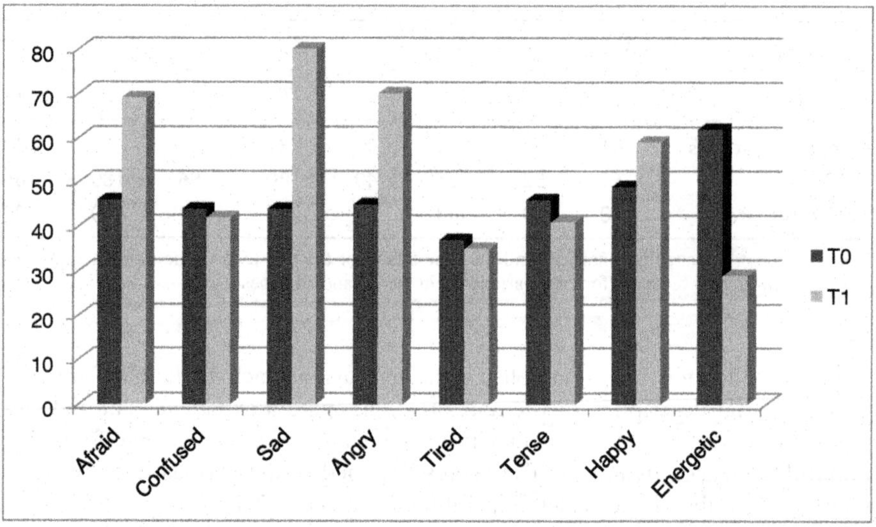

Figure 7.2 M.B. Test scores T0-T1

VAMS; Five Facet; SSQoL; BDI-II; STAI-I; STAI-II; TMA; TMT 1°; TMT 2°

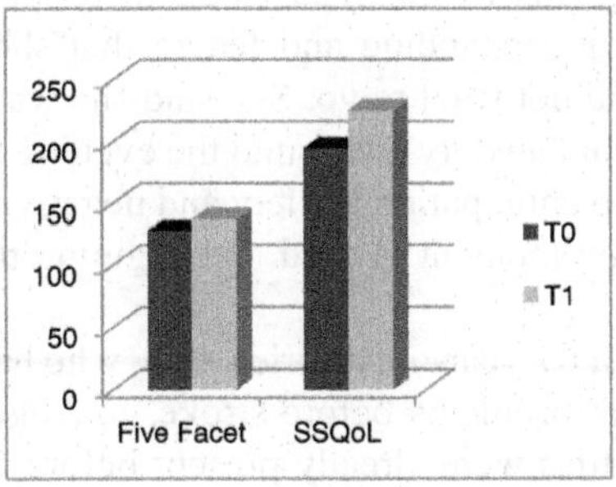

Figure 7.3 M.B. Test scores T0-T1

VAMS; Five Facet; SSQoL; BDI-II; STAI-I; STAI-II; TMA; TMT 1°; TMT 2°

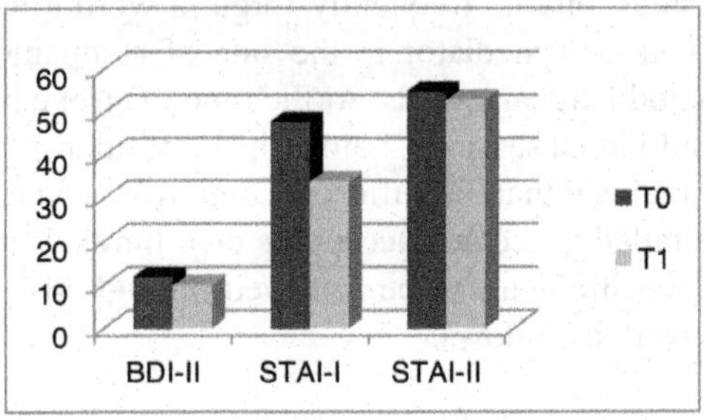

Figure 7.4 M.B. Test scores T0-T1

VAMS; Five Facet; SSQoL; BDI-II; STAI-I; STAI-II; TMA; TMT 1°; TMT 2°

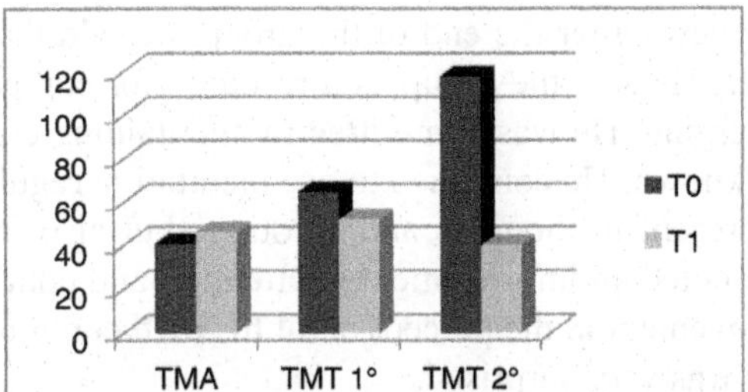

Figure 7.5 M.B. Test scores T0-T1

VAMS; Five Facet; SSQoL; BDI-II; STAI-I; STAI-II; TMA; TMT 1°; TMT 2°

and describe the painful events of her life with detachment and with lower levels of anxiety could help in the problem-solving tasks that she met in work and family life.

From a cognitive point of view, mindfulness-based intervention seemed to have favoured an improvement in attention performance.

During a group session, M.B. talked about an aperitif with colleagues and friends. She was very worried because she had to face a situation in a crowded and noisy public place. This was a situation she had not faced since the stroke. She was afraid of not understanding and feared that she would not be able to communicate, so she did not want to go. She said she was surprised because she faced the situation without anxiety and found the evening relaxing and enjoyable; she had managed to stop anticipation anxiety and negative expectations by trying to be present moment by moment instead of imagining that something negative would happen.

Case: A.F.: A.F. was a 69-year-old married man, who had a son and a daughter. He had important health problems before stroke. In August 2012, he suffered a stroke. Physical difficulties were already present before the stroke; after stroke, movement difficulties and aphasia are added. After functional rehabilitation, he was still able to walk and move. On a linguistic level, he had recovered a lot: he had mild aphasia with circumlocutions and some word substitutions. He often didn't remember names, and he frequently forgot a word after saying it. Before the stroke, he worked as a mediator in the sale of companies. He had a good memory and very good language skills. At the time of stroke he was retired.

He took part in individual sessions, before the mindfulness group. During individual sessions, he realized that his suffering came from changes with stroke and aphasia and that he failed to see and accept his own limits. With the psychologist he identified three specific goals to be achieved through his participation in the group. A.F.'s goals were as follows:

- To stay in a different way in his experience.
- To be more present to himself.
- To use meditation exercises as training to improve attention and concentration.

In individual interviews after the end of the group, he said that the group was a positive experience. He saw the group as a resource for comparison and for the bonds that are emerging. He was committed to maintaining contact and meeting the people he had known. He continued to use meditation regularly.

He was more present in thoughts and emotions but also in the body and in the sensations. He noted an improvement in attention and concentration. He also described an improvement in the perception of his own communication; he felt it more fluid, and he was very surprised.

Overall, a higher level of quality of life was reported which is in line with the improvement in mindfulness skills. The increased ability to observe, act in a conscious way and not to judge his own experience may have contributed to the possibility of entering a different relationship with it and a greater capacity for mental presence, confirming the achievement of his first two goals. The results of the focus training on attention seemed to confirm his subjective feeling also in the attention tests, in particular in the Trail Making Test, showing the direction of change in favour of the achievement of A.F.'s third objective.

The positive change perceived after the intervention and the decision to continue to practice mindfulness confirmed the positive contribution of the group for A.F.

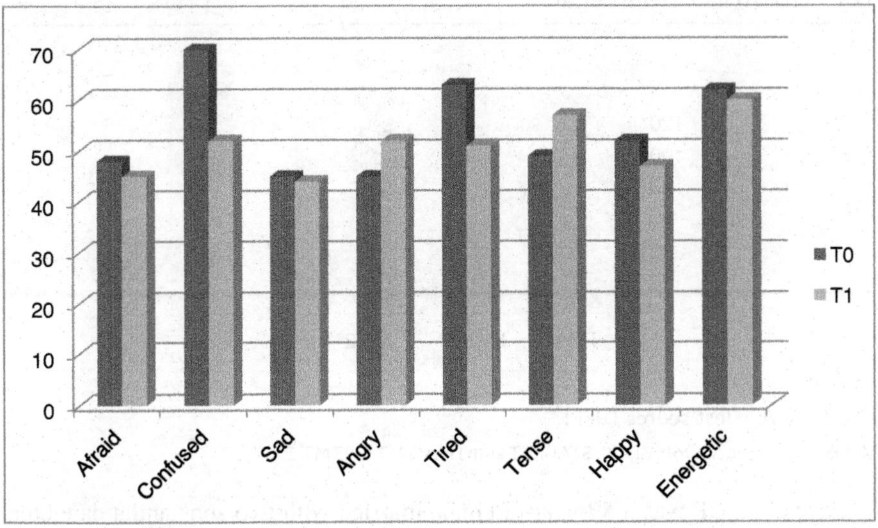

Figure 7.6 A.F. Test scores T0-T1
VAMS; Five Facet; SSQoL; BDI-II; STAI-I; STAI-II; TMA; TMT 1°; TMT 2°

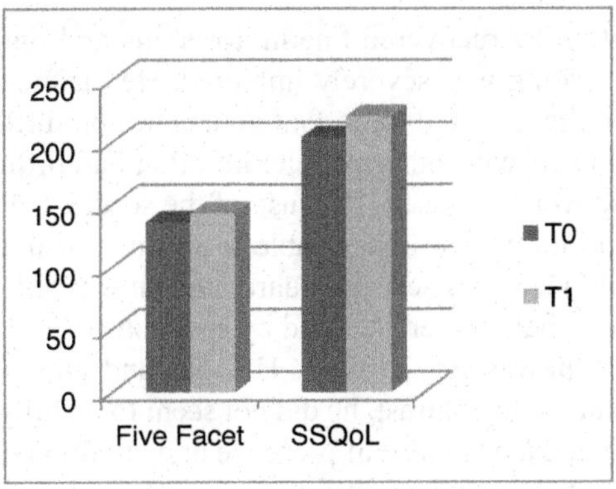

Figure 7.7 A.F. Test scores T0-T1
VAMS; Five Facet; SSQoL; BDI-II; STAI-I; STAI-II; TMA; TMT 1°; TMT 2°

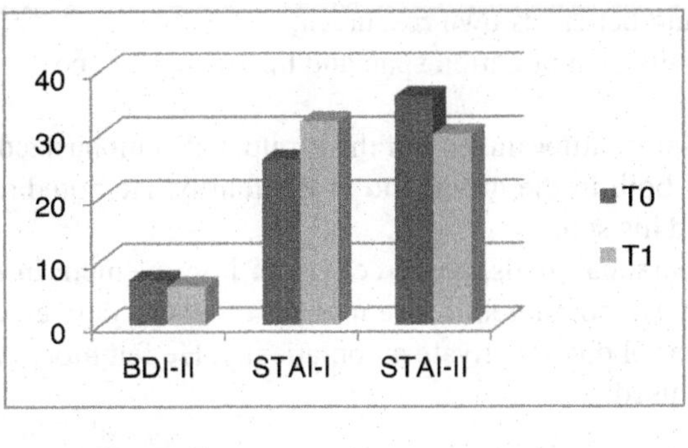

Figure 7.8 A.F. Test scores T0-T1
VAMS; Five Facet; SSQoL; BDI-II; STAI-I; STAI-II; TMA; TMT 1°; TMT 2°

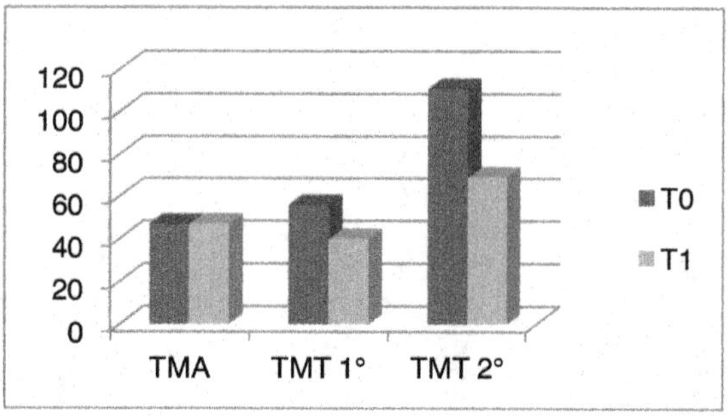

Figure 7.9 A.F. Test scores T0-T1
VAMS; Five Facet; SSQoL; BDI-II; STAI-I; STAI-II; TMA; TMT 1°; TMT 2°

Case C.F.: CF was a 59-year-old man, married with two sons and a daughter. The younger son still lived at home with him and his wife. He lost his job as a result of the stroke and struggled to find new employment. Stroke had already been experienced within the family – his father and his brother had suffered strokes in previous years.

With rehabilitation he recovered fine motor skills and linguistic skills. Aphasia was mild but writing was severely impaired. He claimed to have changed a lot after the stroke; he reported important concentration difficulties and in being able to express himself with other people; he often had difficulty understanding the meaning of the words he used. Because of the stroke, C.F. found his memory abilities worse, and he was no longer able to evaluate situations with clarity as he had done before. He was a security guard, and he was able to assess situations very quickly without being overwhelmed by emotions.

Anger management was very difficult. His wife and sons worried about trigger situations for outbursts. In contrast, he did not seem to be fully aware of his anger. Instead, he recognized a difficulty of presence and attention difficulties.

The goals he wanted to achieve were:

1 To learn more about the situation related to stroke and aphasia and the emotions he experiences;
2 To understand better his own resources;
3 To improve his own attention span and his own presence.

In individual sessions after the end of the group, C.F. emphasized the importance of relationships, both in the group and in the family. He noted a better dialogue with his wife and his sons.

For his own personal goals, he perceived an improvement in recognizing and managing anger. He continued to use meditation every day, especially when he felt that anger was about to activate automatically. He felt more present and more attentive and focused.

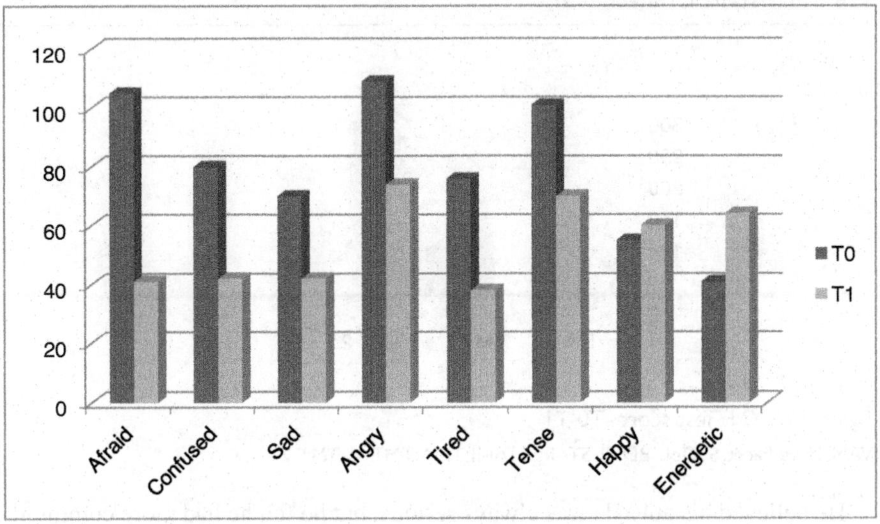

Figure 7.10 C.F. Test scores T0-T1

VAMS; Five Facet; SSQoL; BDI-II; STAI-I; STAI-II; TMA; TMT 1°; TMT 2°

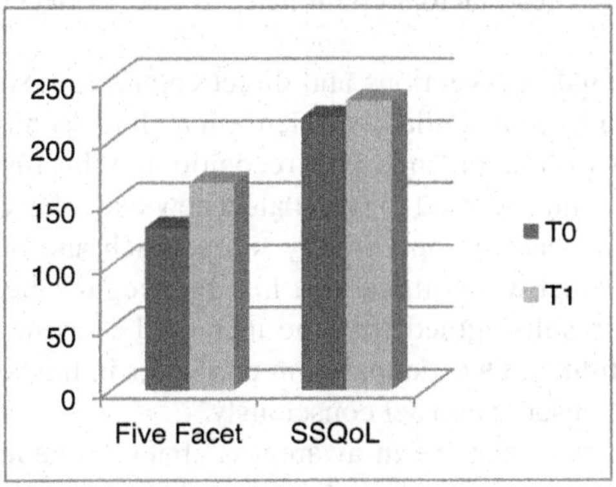

Figure 7.11 C.F. Test scores T0-T1

VAMS; Five Facet; SSQoL; BDI-II; STAI-I; STAI-II; TMA; TMT 1°; TMT 2°

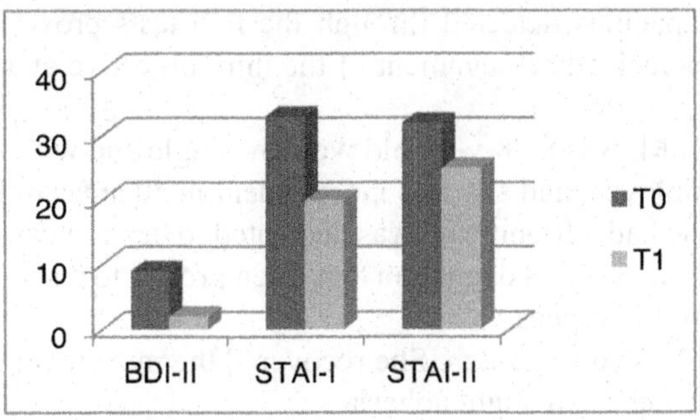

Figure 7.12 C.F. Test scores T0-T1

VAMS; Five Facet; SSQoL; BDI-II; STAI-I; STAI-II; TMA; TMT 1°; TMT 2°

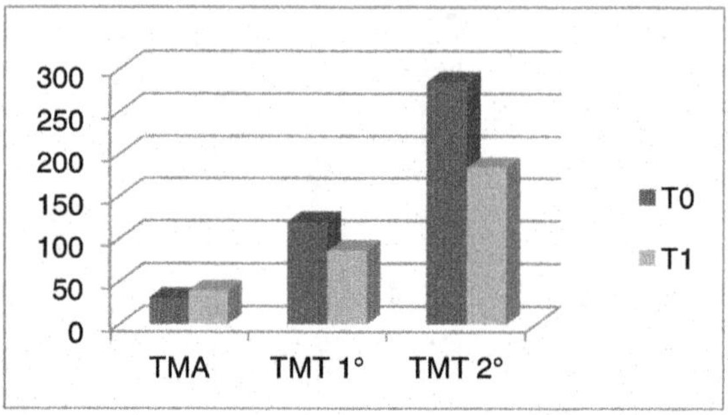

Figure 7.13 C.F. Test scores T0-T1

VAMS; Five Facet; SSQoL; BDI-II; STAI-I; STAI-II; TMA; TMT 1°; TMT 2°

He believed his aphasia was always serious, but he felt he had more communication possibilities.

During the last sessions of group, C.F.'s family and work situation deteriorated; there were tensions with family members, in particular with the son who lived at home with him. These factors could had adversely affected some results over time T1.

Psychoeducational interventions and direct comparison with other group partecipants who had lived a similar experience may have contributed to the understanding of his own situation and to the recognition of his resources.

Mindfulness training seemed to stimulate a new way of accessing his emotions and experience. He had the opportunity to approach and become aware of the emotions of anger that were difficult for him to recognize before participating in the group. These results agreed with the increased awareness detected with the Five Facet Mindfulness Questionnaire, in particular in the components that concern the ability to observe and act consciously.

It was possible that increase in awareness about stroke and aphasia with the increased ability to recognize mental contents may have favored the important decrease in negative emotions, particularly for fear and confusion. Mindfulness training also seemed to have favoured a decrease in anxiety levels. This last effect maybe have contributed both to the emotional level and to the quality of life level.

Attentional capacities detected through the two tests prove to be improved, confirming the perceived achievement of the third objective at a subjective level by C.F.

Case: G.M.: G.M. was a 78-year-old woman, single and without children. She was an office employee, and she was independent in all areas of her life. She liveed alone, and she had a friend who was dedicated to her as a caregiver. She had a relationship with her sister's daughters that often proved to be conflictual because of some personal differences.

She had a stroke two years ago. She recovered the movement even if she soon tired of walking; she had a slight aphasia.

She reported that she had no problem understanding what she felt and what happened to her, but she needed some time to "put things right" with herself.

She had three goals:

- To know and manage the emotions she feels; she doesn't feel adequate and she feels ashamed.
- To learn to slow down, allowing herself to take the right time to listen to others and talk to them.
- To reduce the obsessive thoughts that make her imagine she is in trouble in social communication situations.

A mindfulness-based group could allowed her to get involved in a protected context where she could experience communication and become aware that thoughts are not real facts.

During the individual sessions, after the end of the group, she noted the importance of working with other people.

She expressed a particular relief and sense of calm received from meditation experience, which allowed her to feel more relaxed and to discover in a new way what she felt through the five senses. She continued to practice meditation at home. Furthermore, she claimed to feel more present in life situations. With respect to personal goals, she felt she has reached them at a good level.

G.M.'s first goal was to reduce feelings of shame and inadequacy. From the analysis of the videotapes, several moments emerged in which G.M. had the possibility of 'questioning' some of the convictions she had on the theme of right-wrong: the opening to the debate generated by the experience of mindfulness meditation and the comparison with direct experience of other members of the group on how to live their emotions and thoughts could have given G.M. the possibility of a new look at her mental activity. The judgement theme continued to be a central feature of its functioning. G.M. is in fact linked to 'performance', which is thought to be a pre-morbid characteristic.

Despite these results, it is important to point out that anger, sadness and tension diminished in the mood measures, while happiness increased and the perceived weight of aphasia decreased. State anxiety and trait anxiety were also diminishing, thus suggesting the possible attenuation of dependence on performance judgement.

About her second objective through mindfulness, she seemed to have increased the ability to slow down and give herself time for the commitments that must be completed and in the communication sphere. According to video recordings, the practice of awareness seemed to bring her into a new relationship with her body. In group discussions, she stated that she particularly appreciated body scan; this element could be related to the significant increase in the level of personal care in the test that investigates quality of life (Stroke Specific Quality of Life Scale).

With regard to the third objective, we hypothesize a relationship between the slight decrease in the anxiety indexes (state and trait) detected with the State Trait Anxiety Inventory and brood tendency.

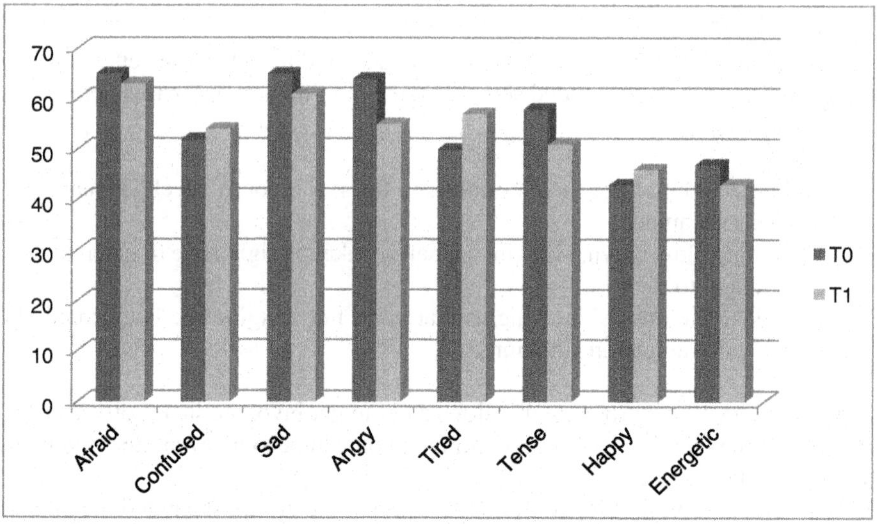

Figure 7.14 M.G. Test scores T0-T1
VAMS; Five Facet; SSQoL; BDI-II; STAI-I; STAI-II; TMA; TMT 1°; TMT 2°

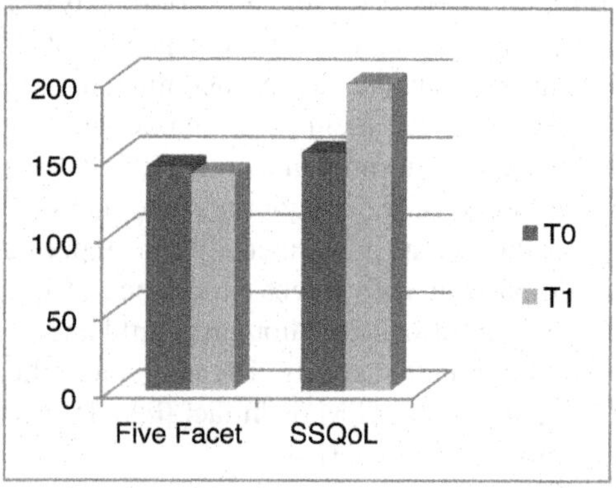

Figure 7.15 M.G. Test scores T0-T1
VAMS; Five Facet; SSQoL; BDI-II; STAI-I; STAI-II; TMA; TMT 1°; TMT 2°

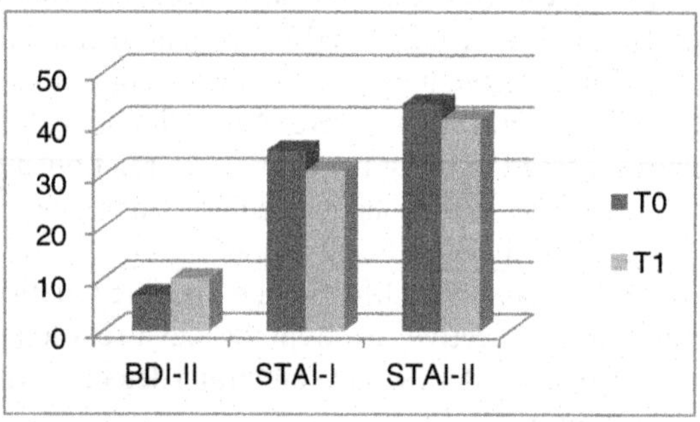

Figure 7.16 M.G. Test scores T0-T1
VAMS; Five Facet; SSQoL; BDI-II; STAI-I; STAI-II; TMA; TMT 1°; TMT 2°

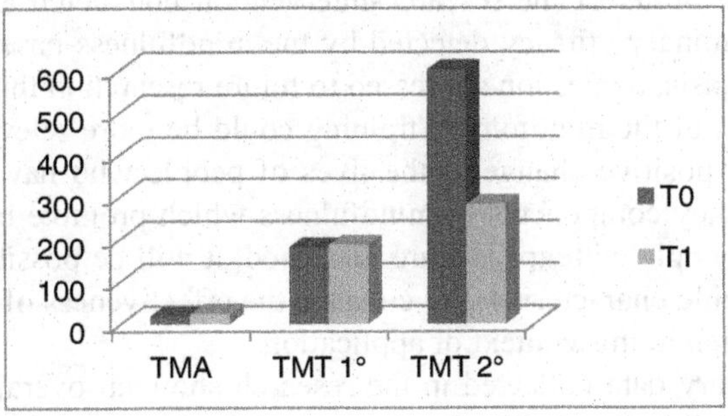

Figure 7.17 M.G. Test scores T0-T1

VAMS; Five Facet; SSQoL; BDI-II; STAI-I; STAI-II; TMA; TMT 1°; TMT 2°

Compared with the other participants, the results of G.M. taken from the FFMQ and SS-QoL do not go in the same direction. An improvement in the quality of life is reported; however, there is a worsening in mindfulness skills. Considering that G.M. seemed in general to have a high level of communication impairment with respect to the other components, the comparison of the results related to the FFMQ and SS-QOL tests would seem to suggest a possible inadequacy of the first tool for mindfulness abilities in aphasia.

Overall reflections on the group data: From the qualitative analysis of the video recordings of the group and from the moment of individual restitution, two reflections emerge in the direction of the treatment objective.

All mindfulness group participants report that they have experienced the importance of interpersonal relationships and the effective possibility of meeting people and participating in social activities, starting from those proposed by the CIRP Aphasia Center. As a research-intervention, the object of investigation is constituted by the potentialities and the limits of the treatment, in order to offer guidelines for future interventions in the field of psychological support for people with aphasia. The choice of the small group is considered justified by the context of application: it is considered the ideal condition for an emancipation space among people who have a communication deficit.

This is research in the absence of a control group. Therefore, it is not possible to attribute with certainty the change to the mindfulness intervention. The preliminary results are also not generalizable to the potential efficacy of mindfulness-based treatment in cases of aphasia since only people with production aphasia and mild linguistic impairment were included in the group.

Although the research does not present an analysis of the significance of the results and the data of the follow-up, the preliminary data obtained are encouraging as they go in the hypothesized direction, highlighting an improvement in the quality of life and a strengthening of interpersonal relationships.

Regarding mindfulness, it has been argued that specific training components may play a more relevant role in some application contexts than others.

Aware of the limits of the research-intervention conducted and the need to verify the preliminary efficacy detected by the mindfulness-based treatment for people with aphasia, a question addressed to future research in this area emerges. Which elements of the mindfulness training could be more relevant than others in generating a positive change in the lives of people who have gone through aphasia? If the key components of mindfulness which promote better wellbeing conditions for people with aphasia are identified, it will be possible to construct a tool with specific characteristics to enhance the effectiveness of a mindfulness-based intervention in this context of application.

The preliminary data collected in the research show an overall improvement in the quality of life detected in the Stroke Specific Quality of Life scale in the re-test phase. In general, the indices for the detection of depression and anxiety symptoms agree with the detection of the level of the quality of life of the group, reflecting the decrease in symptoms of anxiety and depression.

From direct comparison of the participants of the mindfulness group, it is also observed the importance that the comparison with other people and the sharing of the meaning of a painful experience, such as that of aphasia, has had for each of them.

A future challenge could be to identify which components of an intervention based on mindfulness could favour more than others a change in the direction of the wellbeing of the person with aphasia.

A consideration on the possible inadequacy of the instrument for the measurement of mindfulness in cases of people with aphasia was conducted, we hypothesize that test structure is too difficult to understand for person with communication impairment. In other contexts, where there is no linguistic compromise, a feasible way could be to use the Five Facet Mindfulness Questionnaire, with which it is possible to measure individually the five components identified at the base of the mindfulness skill. In the specific case of aphasia, precisely in relation to the problems highlighted in the use of the instrument, this does not seem an easy path to undertake.

Conclusions

This paper has presented two tentative sources of preliminary evidence to support the rationale for using mindfulness interventions for people with aphasia. A detailed descriptive case study was presented initially to illustrate in detail how a mindfulness intervention can affect emotional functioning and quality of life for a survivor. Then the preliminary results of a small mindfulness for aphasia group are shared. While this data has not been subjected to any single-case quantitative analyses, the trends in improvements on measures of both mood and cognitive changes in higher control of attentional processes are evident and warrant future rigorous research to substantiate. Generalizations about gender differences are not possible to make because of the small sample size. These data are tentatively supportive of the effectiveness of mindfulness group intervention in fostering a different relationship with one's own experience.

In particular, it is thought that these interventions may have contributed the following for people with aphasia: training the ability to focus on one's own experience (on a bodily, emotional and thought level), together with the increased capacity of awareness and decentralization with respect to one's own mental contents.

Moreover, it is hypothesized that the lower levels of anxiety may be a consequence of the practice of mindfulness and that this effect can in turn act as an intermediary on the improvement detected in the quality-of-life level.

More research in this clinical context is needed to establish with more certainty, through the further administration of the treatment and the inclusion of control groups, the advanced efficacy based on the data of the present intervention research.

Note

1 Maristella Crielesi, psychologist, psychotherapist, mindfulness teacher. CIRP – Creare Integrazione Resilienza Possibilità – Centro Afasia, Torino, Italy. Contact: maristella.crielesi@cirpafasia.it

Bibliography

Amadei, G. (2013). *Mindfulness. Essere consapevoli*. Bologna: Il Mulino.

Arruda, J. E., Stern, R. A., & Somerville, J. A. (1999). Measurement of mood states in stroke patients: Validation of the visual analog mood scales. *Archives of Physical Medicine and Rehabilitation, 80*(6), 676–680.

Ashworth, F., Gracey, F., & Gilbert, P. (2011). Compassion focused therapy after traumatic brain injury: Theoretical foundations and a case illustration. *Brain Impairment, 12*(2), 128–139.

Baer, R. A. (A cura di). (2010). *Assessing mindfulness and acceptance processes in clients*. Oakland: New Harbinger Publications. Trad. it.

Baer, R. A., Smith, G. T., & Allen, K. B. (2004). Assessment of mindfulness by self report: The Kentucky inventory of mindfulness skills. *Assessment, 11*(3), 191–206.

Baer, R. A., Smith, G. T., Hopkins, J., Krietemeyer, J., & Toney, L. (2006). Using self-report assessment methods to explore facets of mindfulness. *Assessment, 13*, 27–45.

Bar, M. (2007). The proactive brain: Using analogies and associations to generate predictions. *Trends in Cognitive Sciences, 11*(9), 280–289.

Bara, B. (1999). *Pragmatica cognitiva. I processi mentali della comunicazione*. Torino: Bollati Boringhieri.

Bartha, L., & Benke, T. (2003). Acute conduction aphasia: An analysis of 20 cases. *Brain and Language, 85*, 93–108.

Beck, A. T., Steer, R. A., & Brown, G. K. (A cura di). (1996). *BDI-II Beck Depression Inventory-II*. Firenze: Giunti, 2006.

Bédard, M., Felteau, M., Marshall, S., Dubois, S., Gibbons, C., Klein, R., & Weaver, B. (2012). Mindfulness-based cognitive therapy: Benefits in reducing depression following a traumatic brain injury. *Advances Spring, 26*(1), 14–20.

Bédard, M., Felteau, M., Mazmanian, D., Fedyk, K., Klein, R., Richardson, J. . . . Minthorn-Biggs, M. B. (2003). Pilot evaluation of a mindfulness-based intervention to improve

quality of life among individuals who sustained traumatic brain injuries. *Disability and Rehabilitation, 25*(13), 722–731.
Brown, K. W., & Ryan, R. M. (2003). The benefits of being present: Mindfulness and its role in psychological well-being. *Journal of Personality and Social Psychology, 84*(4), 822–848.
Cardaciotto, L. A., Herbert, J. D., Forman, E. M., Moitra, E., & Farrow, V. (2007). The assessment of present-moment awareness and acceptance: The Philadelphia Mindfulness Scale. *Assessment, 15*, 204–223.
Cardano, M. (2011). *La ricerca qualitativa*. Bologna: Il Mulino.
Chadwick, P., Hember, M., Symes, J., Peters, E., Kuipers, E., & Dagnan, D. (2008). Responding mindfully to unpleasant thoughts and images: Reliability and validity of the Southampton Mindfulness Questionnaire (SMQ). *British Journal of Clinical Psychology, 47*(4), 451–455.
Chapey, R. (2001). *Language intervention strategies in aphasia and related neurogenic communication disorders*. Philadelphia, PA: Lippincott Williams & Wilkins.
Chau, J. P. C., Thompson, D. R., Twinn, S., Chang, A. M., & Woo, J. (2009). Determinants of participation restriction among community dwelling stroke survivors: A path analysis. *BMC Neurology, 9*, 49.
Christopher, M. S., Christopher, V., & Charoensuk, S. (2009). Assessing "western" mindfulness among Thai Theravāda Buddhist Monks. *Mental Health, Religion & Culture, 12*(3), 303–314.
Conze, E. (1955). *Buddhism its essence and development*. New York, NY: Dover Publications.
Damasio, A. R. (1992). Aphasia. *The New England Journal of Medicine, 326*(8), 531–539.
Davids, T. W. R., & Stede, W. (1921–1925). *Pali-English dictionary*. The Pali Text Society's.
DeRubeis, R., Gelfand, L., Tang, T., & Simons, A. (1999). Medication versus cognitive behavior therapy for severely depressed out patients: Megaanalysis of four randomized comparisons. *American Journal of Psychiatry, 156*(7), 1007–1013.
Dickinson, J., Friary, P., & McCann, C. M. (2017). The influence of mindfulness meditation on communication and anxiety: A case study of a person with aphasia. *Aphasiology, 31*(9), 1044–1058.
Didonna, F. (2008). *Clinical handbook of mindfulness*. New York: Springer.
Didonna, F., & Bosio, V. (2012). Assessing mindfulness skills: A validation study of the Italian version of the Five Facet Mindfulness Questionnaire. *Psicoterapia Cognitiva e Comportamentale, 8*(3), 261–284.
Ellis-Hill, C. S., & Horn, S. (2000). Change in identity and self-concept: A new theoretical approach to recovery following a stroke. *Clinical Rehabilitation, 14*(3), 279–287.
Feigin, V. L., Lawes, C. M. M., Bennett, D. A., & Anderson, C. S. (2003). Stroke epidemiology: A review of population-based studies of incidence, prevalence, and case-fatality in the late 20th century. *Stroke Epidemiology, 2*(1), 43–53.
Feldman, G., Hayes, A., Kumar, S., Greeson, J., & Laurenceau, J. P. (2007). Mindfulness and emotion regulation: The development and initial validation of the Cognitive and Affective Mindfulness Scale-Revised (CAMS-R). *Journal Psychopatolology and Behavioral Assessment, 26*, 177–190.
Filoramo, G. (A cura di). (1996). *Storia delle religioni. Vol. 4 Religioni dell'India e dell'Estremo Oriente*. Roma-Bari: Gius. Laterza.
Folstein, M. F., Maiberger, R., & McHugh, P. R. (1977). Mood disorder as a specific complication of stroke. *Journal of Neurology Neurosurgery and Psychiatry, 40*, 1018–1020.
Frühwald, S., Löffler, H., Eher, R., Saletu, B., & Baumhackl, U. (2001). Relationship between depression, anxiety and quality of life: A study of stroke patients compared to chronic low back pain and myocardial ischemia patients. *Psychopathology, 34*, 50–56.

Gainotti, G. (1997). Emotional, psychological e psychosocial problems of aphasic patients: An introduction. *Aphasiology, 11*(7), 635–650.

Gainotti, G., Antonucci, G., Marra, C., & Paolucci, S. (2001). Relation between depression after stroke, antidepressant therapy, and functional recovery. *Journal of Neurology Neurosurgery and Psychiatry, 71*, 258–261.

Gilbert, P., & Procter, S. (2006). Compassionate mind training for people with high shame and self-criticism: Overview and pilot study of a group therapy approach. *Clinical Psychology and Psychotherapy, 13*, 353–379.

Giommi, F. (2005). Il potere dell'attenzione: la prospettiva della mindfulness. In B. Bara (a cura di), *Nuovo manuale di psicoterapia cognitiva* (pp. 231–258). Torino: Bollati Boringhieri.

Giovagnoli, A. R., Del Pesce, M., Mascheroni, S., Simoncelli, M., Laiacona, M., & Capitani, E. (1996). Trail Making Test: Normative values from 287 normal adult controls. *Italian Journal of Neurological Science, 17*(4), 305–309.

Gloaguen, V., Cottraux, J., Cucherat, M., & Blackburn, I. (1998). A meta-analysis of the effects of cognitive therapy in depressed patients. *Journal of Affective Disorders, 49*(1), 59–72.

Grossman, P., Niemann, L., Schmidt, S., & Walach, H. (2004). Mindfulness-based stress reduction and health benefits. A meta-analysis. *Journal of Psychosomatic Research, 57*, 35–43.

Hackett, M. L., & Anderson, C. S. (2005). Predictors of depression after stroke: A systematic review of observational studies. *Stroke, 36*(10), 2296–2301.

Hackett, M. L., Yapa, C., Parag, V., & Anderson, C. S. (2005). Frequency of depression after stroke. A systematic review of observational studies. *American Heart Association, 36*, 1330–1340.

Hilari, K. (2011). The impact of stroke: Are people with aphasia different to those without? *Disability and Rehabilitation, 33*(3), 211–218.

Hochstenbach, J. (2000). Rehabilitation is more than functional recovery. *Disability and Rehabilitation, 22*(4), 201–204.

Jacobson, N. S., & Hollon, S. D. (1996). Cognitive-behavior therapy versus pharmacotherapy: Now that the jury's returned its verdict, it's time to present the rest of the evidence. *Journal of Consulting and Clinical Psychology, 64*(1), 74–80.

Jha, A. P., Krompinger, J., & Baime, M. J. (2007). Mindfulness training modifies subsystems of attention. *Cognitive Affective and Behavioral Neurosciences, 7*(2), 109–119.

Kabat-Zinn, J. (1996). Mindfulness: cos'è e cosa non è e il suo ruolo nell'assistenza sanitaria e nella medicina. In Y. Haruki, Y. Ishii, & M. Suzuki (Eds.), *Comparative and psychological study of meditation*. Netherlands: Eburon.

Kabat-Zinn, J. (2003). Mindfulness-based interventions in context: Past, present, and future. *Clinical Psychology: Science and Practice, 10*(2), 144–156.

Kabat-Zinn, J., Lipworth, L., & Burney, R. (1984). The clinical use of mindfulness meditation for the self-regulation of chronic pain. *Journal of Biobehavioral Medicine, 8*(2), 163–190.

Kabat-Zinn, J., Massion, A. O., Kristeller, J., Peterson, L. G., Fletcher, K. E., Pbert, L. . . . Santorelli, S. F. (1992). Effectiveness of a meditation-based stress reduction program in the treatment of anxiety disorders. *American Journal of Psychiatry, 149*, 936–943.

Kabat-Zinn, J., Wheeler, E., Light, T., Skillings, A., Scharf, M., Cropley, T. . . . Bernhard, J. (1998). Influence of a mindfulness meditation-based stress reduction intervention on rates of skin clearing in patients with moderate to severe psoriasis Undergoing Photo

Therapy (UVB) and Photochemotherapy (PUVA). *Journal of Biobehavioral Medicine, 60*(5), 625–632.
Kagan, A. (1998). Supported conversation for adults with aphasia: Methods and resources for training conversation partners. *Aphasiology, 12*(9), 816–830.
Kauhanen, M. L., Korpelainen, J. T., Hiltunen, P., Nieminen, P., Sotaniemi, K. A., & Myllylä, V. V. (2000). Domains and determinants of quality of life after stroke caused by brain infarction. *Archives of Physical Medicine and Rehabilitation, 81*(12), 1541–1546.
Kenneth, G., & Steven, A. (2010). Compassion focused therapy for eating disorders. International *Journal of Cognitive Therapy, 3*(Special Section: Compassion Focused Therapy), 141–158.
Làdavas, E., & Berti, A. (2002). *Neuropsicologia*. Bologna: Il Mulino.
Laures-Gore, J., & Marshall, R. S. (2016). Mindfulness meditation in aphasia: a case report. *NeuroRehabilitation, 38*, 321–329.
Linehan, M. M., Comtois, K. A., Murray, A. M., Brown, M. Z., Gallop, R. J., Heard, H. L. . . . Lindenboim, N. (2006). Two-year randomized controlled trial and follow-up of dialectical behavior therapy vs therapy by expert for suicidal behaviors and borderline personality disorder. *Archives of General Psychiatry, 63*(7), 757–766.
Marshall, R. S., Laures-Gore, J., & Love, K. (2018). Brief mindfulness meditation group training in aphasia: Exploring attention, language and psychophysiological outcomes. *International Journal of Language & Communication Disorders, 53*(1), 40–54.
Mayo, N. E., Wood-Dauphinee S., Côté, R., Durcan, L., & Carlton, J. (2002). Activity, participation, and quality of life 6 months poststroke. *Archives of Physical Medicine and Rehabilitation, 83*, 1035–1042.
Mazzucchi, A. (a cura di). (2011). *La riabilitazione neuropsicologica. Premesse teoriche e applicazioni cliniche*. Milano: Elsevier Srl.
Monte, S., Crielesi, M., Di Pietro, M., & Muò, R. (2015). *Il gruppo operativo "Conversazione Narrativa": impostazione di una ricerca e di un intervento psicoterapeutico con persone afasiche*. Gruppi, 2015 Fascicolo 1, Milan: Franco Angeli Editore.
Moustgaard, A., Bedard, M., & Felteau, M. (2007). Mindfulness-based Cognitive Therapy (MBCT) for individuals who had a stroke: Results from a Pilot 90 Study. *The Journal of Cognitive Rehabilitation, 25*(4), 4–10.
Nelken, I. (2012). Predictive information processing in the brain: The neural perspective. *International Journal of Psychophysiology, 83*, 253–255.
Orenstein, E., Basilakos, A., & Shisler Marshall, R. (2012). Effects of mindfulness meditation on three individuals with aphasia. *International Journal of Language & Communication Disorders/Royal College of Speech & Language Therapists, 47*(6), 673–684. https://doi.org/10.1111/j.1460-6984.2012.00173.x
Parr, S., Byng, S., Gilpin, S., & Ireland, C. (1997). *Talking about aphasia: Living with loss of language after stroke*. Buckingham: Oxford University Press.
Pedon, A., & Gnisci, A. (2004). *Metodologia della ricerca psicologica*. Bologna: Il Mulino.
Percheron, M. (1956). *Le bouddha et le Bouddhisme*. Paris: Seuil.
Petrocchi, N., & Couyoumdjian, A. (2012). L'impiego delle tecniche della terapia focalizzata sulla compassione per promuovere il processo di accettazione in psicoterapia. *Cognitivismo Clinico, 9*(2), 178–190.
Sacco, S., Stracci, F., Cerone, D., Ricci, S., & Carolei, A. (2011). Epidemiology of stroke in Italy. *International Journal of Stroke, 6*, 219–227.
Segal, Z. V., Williams, J. M., & Teasdale, J. D. (2001). *Mindfulness-based cognitive therapy for depression: A new approach to preventing relapse*. New York: Guilford Press.

Siegel, D. J. (2007). *The mindful brain*. Los Angeles, CA: Mind Your Brain Inc.

Speca, M., Carlson, L., Goodey, E., & Angen, M. (2000). A randomized, wait-list controlled clinical trial: The effect of a mindfulness meditation-based stress reduction program on mood and symptoms of stress in cancer outpatients. *Journal of Biobehavioral Medicine*, *62*(5), 613–622.

Spielberger, C. D. (1968). *The State-Trait Anxiety Inventory (S T A I): Test manual for form X*. Washington, DC: Consulting Psychologists Press.

Spinnler, H., & Tognoni, G. (1987). Standardizzazione e Taratura Italiana si Test Neuropsicologici. *The Italian Journal of Neurological Sciences*, *6*(Supplement 8), 47–50.

Sutcliffe, L. M., & Lincoln, N. B. (1998). The assessment of depression in aphasic stroke patients: The development of the Stroke Aphasic Depression Questionnaire. *Clinical Rehabilitation*, *12*(6), 506–513. 91.

Teasdale, J. D., Segal, Z. V., & Williams, J. M. G. (2003). Mindfulness training and problem formulation. *Clinical Psychology: Science and Practice*, *10*(2), 157–160.

Trainor, L. J. (2012). Predictive information processing is a fundamental learning mechanism present in early development: Evidence from infants. *International Journal of Psychophysiology*, *83*, 256–258.

Tse, P. U., Rivest, J., Intriligator, J., & Canavagh, P. (2004). Attention and the subjective expansion of time. *Percept Psychophys*, *66*, 1171–1189.

Valentine, E. R., & Sweet, P. L. G. (1999). Meditation and attention: A comparison of the effects of concentrative and mindfulness meditation on sustained attention. *Mental Health, Religion and Culture*, *2*(1), 59–70.

Walach, H., Buchheld, N., Buttenmüller, V., Kleinknecht, N., & Schmidt, S. (2006). Measuring mindfulness – The Freiburg Mindfulness Inventory (FMI). *Personality and Individual Differences*, *40*(8), 1543–1555.

Walsh, R., & Roche, L. (1979). Precipitation of acute psychotic episodes by intensive meditation in individuals with a hystory of schizophrenia. *American Journal of Psychiatry*, *136*(8), 1085–1086.

Warlow, C. P. (1998). Epidemiology of stroke. *The Lancet*, *352*, SIII 1–4.

Welstein, N., Brown, K. W., & Ryan, R. M. (2008). A multi-method examination of the effects of mindfulness on stress attribution, coping, and emotional wellbeing. *Journal of Research in Personality*, *43*, 374–385.

Whisman, M. A., Perez, J. E., & Ramel, W. (2000). Factor structure of the Beck Depression Inventory – Second Edition (BDI-II) in a student sample. *Journal of Clinical Psychology*, *56*(4), 545–551.

Williams, L. S., Weinberger, M., Harris, L. E., Clark, D. O., & Biller, J. (1999). Development of a stroke-s quality of life scale. *Stroke*, *30*(7), 1362–1369.

World Health Organization. (2011). *World report on disability*. Geneva: World Health Organization.

Chapter 8

The potential contribution of mind-body interventions within psychological support following aphasia

A conceptual review and case study

Giles N. Yeates[1]

Psychological needs and aphasia in acquired neurological conditions

The presence of communication difficulties (restrictions in expression and comprehension of language categorised within the typology of aphasias and related impairments) in acquired neurological conditions such as stroke and traumatic brain injury is associated with poorer mental health outcomes, such as anxiety (Menlove et al., 2015), depression (Baker et al., 2018; Kauhenan et al., 199; Kutlubaev & Hackett, 2014), frustration, hopelessness, disruptions to sense of self, social isolation and reduced wellbeing (e.g., Cruice, Hill, Worrall, & Hickson, 2010; Hilari, Needle, & Harrison, 2012; Parr, 2001; Shadden, 2005).

Importantly for this article, these emotional needs, interconnected with communication restrictions, also commonly co-occur with physical impairments (e.g., commonly full hemiparesis or restricted mobility/sensation of the right side of the body following a left middle cerebral artery infarction, and/or wider problems with balance and gait) and cognitive impairments that are independent from the aphasia (difficulties in aspects of attention, visuo-spatial abilities, and planning and organisation). Interventions delivered to provide emotional support need to be also situated within this wider array of needs, and the social restrictions (participation, isolation) that can emerge as a result.

Professional and linguistic limitations in neuro-rehabilitation interventions

The complexity and interconnected, multi-domain nature of post-injury difficulties require innovative options of support that address body, mind (with all of its unique forms of disturbance in ABI) and social relationships, without high demands for linguistic expression and comprehension for clients. However, forms of support commonly offered in ABI services are often demarcated and punctuated by professional boundaries, and are time limited. As a result, physiotherapy interventions can be compromised by the impact of cognitive difficulties (e.g., initiation and/or memory) and emotional influences (low mood, anxiety). Survivors themselves often prioritise a need for continued physiotherapy beyond the time limits of public service provision rather than seek psychological support, despite others around them identifying survivor adjustment needs.

Traditional paradigms of psychological therapy dominate ABI services' provision of emotional support for survivors. Common orientations such as cognitive behavioural Therapy (Gracey et al., 2015), psychodynamic (Solms & Kaplan-Solms, 2002) and systemic (Bowen, Yeates & Palmer, 2010) are supported by adjunctive cognitive rehabilitation strategies and technological adaptations (Yeates, 2014) to mitigate the potentially negative impact of cognitive difficulties on therapy outcome (e.g., Yeates et al., 2008). However, all of these are based on the traditional, seated, talking-therapy format. A ubiquitous seated verbal exchange for an hour is not a sufficiently flexible and innovative response to the myriad of survivors' altered relationships with their minds post injury. Even before aphasia is considered, cognitive difficulties such as working memory and attentional and executive impairments can result in a restricted ability to manage the content of one's mind, even to access positive/alternative thoughts, and exceptions to adversarial life events, as required by many therapy orientations. Attentional/arousal difficulties may mean it is hard for a survivor to focus on a set of ideas while sat down in conversation for an hour (as would barriers to seating arising from physical disability).

The presence of communication difficulties such as aphasia may preclude the reliance of a conversational-based form of emotional support altogether. In recognising the uncertainty of the effectiveness of talking therapies for people with aphasia, many clinicians do not attempt such intervention, and as a result, survivors are left without any form of emotional support whatsoever (Dalemans, Wade, van den Heuvel, & de Witte, 2009). These specific omissions co-occur alongside common neglected areas of support for all survivors of acquired brain injury (ABI). A direct engagement with dimensions of spirituality and existential meaning are commonly omitted from psychology sessions (and those of other rehabilitation professionals, Yeates, in press a). Finally, the social isolation that characterises survivors' longer-term trajectories is insufficiently addressed by time-limited psychosocial intervention (Behn et al., 2018), mirrored by a range of barriers to survivors' satisfactory access to community leisure and social resources for the general population. This is despite the demonstration of the value of multiple, long-term, social group membership for survivor post-injury identity (Haslam et al., 2008).

There is a general need, therefore, for interventions that simultaneously address mind and body of all survivors: physical, cognitive and emotional needs, alongside acknowledging the enduring nature of these difficulties and the wider context of social isolation. Within this, there is a specific need for new paradigms of emotional support that are less reliant on verbal mediums to respond to these needs following aphasia. Clinicians working with neurological patients across different service contexts have looked beyond talking therapy paradigms to find novel and flexible approaches to emotional and existential support that may adequately respond to the aforementioned diversity and complexity. To this end, Eastern spiritual, philosophical and health cultivation practices have become increasingly accessed as a resource.

Eastern mind-body practices in neuro-rehabilitation

Asian spiritual traditions are both ancient and diverse, operationalising different ideas of the mind and spirit. One common thread running through the three traditions that have influenced published neuro-rehabilitation work to date – mindfulness, yoga and tai chi – is a focus on using the body to manage the mind and create opportunities for spiritual growth. As such, the approach to mind and the specific mind-body practices from each offer new opportunities to survivors of ABI in managing emotional and existential challenges (Yeates, 2015, in press a, in press b; Yeates & Farrell, 2014, 2018).

Mindfulness approaches

Mindfulness and non-judgemental relationship to mental events and desires, concepts and practices derived from Buddhist ideas (Kabat-Zinn, 2003), have been applied widely within Western psychotherapy and health settings, including in neurological services with people diagnosed with Parkinson's disease (Advocat et al., 2016; Cash, Ekouevi, Kilbourn, & Lageman, 2015; Dissanayaka et al., 2016; Fitzpatrick, Simpson, & Smith, 2010; Pickut et al., 2013, 2015); multiple sclerosis (Aghabagheri, Mohammadkhani, Omrani, & Farahmand, 2012; Blankespoor, Schellekens, Vos, Speckens, & de Jong, 2017; Bogosian et al., 2015; Bogosian, Hughes, Norton, Silber, & Moss-Morris, 2016; Grossman et al., 2010; Hoogerwerf, Bol, Lobbestael, Hupperts, & van Heugten, 2017; Kolahkaj & Zargar, 2015; Senders, Bourdette, Hanes, Vijaysgree, & Shinto, 2014; Simpson et al., 2014; Simpson, Mair, & Mercer, 2017; Simpson, Byrne, Wood, Mair, & Mercer, 2018); epilepsy (Tang, Poon, & Kwan, 2015; Thompson et al., 2015) and acquired brain injury subtypes such as traumatic brain injury and stroke where communication difficulties do not characterise the sample (Bedard et al., 2003, 2005, 2012; Detert, in press; Detert & Douglas, 2014; and mixed neurological sample Johansson, Bjhur, & Rönnbäck, 2012; Kenuk & Porter, 2017; McHugh & Wood, 2013; McMillan, Robertson, Brock, & Chorlton, 2002; Moustgaard, Bedard, & Felteau, 2007). Aspects of bodily experience such as awareness of the breath during sitting meditation can be used as a stimulus to detach from mental contents. Mindfulness is also a key element of increasingly popular acceptance and commitment therapy interventions in neuro-rehabilitation (Todd & Smith, in press; Whiting, Simpson, Ciarrochi, & McLeod, 2012). Psychotherapy interventions using a mindfulness framework focus on helping the survivor detach or decouple from distressing mental events, often using their body or breath, to work towards a compassionate, non-judgemental position on their experiences. From a technical neuropsychotherapy perspective (i.e., the field of adapting psychological therapies in response to cognitive difficulties in neurological conditions), the aim to decouple from negative mental phenomena rather than actively try and access alternative psychological perspectives is more accessible to many survivors.

In an attempt to widen the accessibility of mindfulness practices to those who would struggle solely with seated meditation (the main vehicle of mindfulness practice in the majority of clinical interventions), some clinicians have used martial arts movements to create new interventions for those with complex needs, and have considered the value of such for people with neurological conditions (Russell, 2011; Russell & Tatton-Ramos, 2014).

Yoga

There is a considerable appeal of approaches that involve the body more centrally in meditative practice and so offer additional clinical gains such as increased balance, postural control, mobility, strength and flexibility, and so can simultaneously contribute to both physical and psychological goals post injury. Yoga means 'yoke' or 'union', a system of different meditative and lifestyle practices from the Indian subcontinent, and is intertwined with the Vedic tradition and Hinduism. One of eight strands of yoga that is most commonly associated with the name is the practice of *asana*, or adopting physical poses (that work the practitioner's flexibility, balance and strength) while simultaneously regulating the breath and focusing the mind.

The application of yoga in a neuro-rehabilitation setting has been described in several reviews and individual studies of stroke survivors (Bastille & Gill-Body, 2004; Lazaridou, Philbrook, & Tzika, 2013; Lynton, Kligler, & Shiflett, 2007), reporting gains in physical and cognitive functioning alongside reduction in stress. Yogic movements have traditionally been included in mindfulness-based stress reduction protocols with neurological patients, such as in a stroke study by Moustgaard et al. (2007). Donnelly, Linnea, Grant, and Lichtenstein (2014) demonstrated the feasibility of a yoga intervention for survivors of traumatic brain injury, plus reporting indications of benefits in aspects of quality of life relative to a control group. Yeates and colleagues (2014) demonstrated gains in the reduction of anxiety and fatigue across survivors in their single-case analysis of a pilot yoga group within a community brain injury service, and gains in respiratory, physical and psychological functioning have been reported in a pilot by Silverthorne, Khalsa, Gueth, DeAvilla, and Pansini (2012). Detailed brain injury case study accounts have been provided by Shravat (2014) and Schmid, Miller, Van Puymbroeck, and Schalk (2016).

Participants with epilepsy were found to benefit from yoga plus acceptance and commitment therapy (Lundgren, Dahl, Yardi, & Melin, 2008) and a yoga/meditation protocol (Rajesh, Jayachandran, Mohandas, & Radhakrishnan, 2006), with gains, including reduced seizure frequency and increased quality of life.

Systematic reviews have been conducted for yoga studies with progressive neurological disorders. Roland (2014) notes modest gains reported across studies of participants with Parkinson's disease, in outcomes including functional mobility, balance, lower limb strength, upper and lower flexibility, mood and sleep. Roland inferred that these findings have positive implications for gait, postural stability, balance confidence, rigidity, shuffling gait and flexed posture. Well-designed future studies are required to strengthen these findings. In the multiple sclerosis literature, Cramer, Lauche, Azizi, Dobos, and Langhorst (2014) found evidence across studies for the benefits of yoga on fatigue and mood, but not health-related quality of life, physical or cognitive functioning. They concluded, however, that the evidence for yoga in multiple sclerosis was insufficiently robust to make clinical recommendations.

Following the suggestions by Russell (2011) that the body can be more centrally incorporated into meditative practice to widen the accessibility of such practices to service users who struggle with attention, these yoga interventions within neuro-rehabilitation offer both new paradigms for emotional support and concurrent physical gains too. In relation to spiritual care, the aforementioned survivor experience of fragmentation may be uniquely approached by the aim in yogic asana practice of unifying mind, body and spirit in an embodied meditative tradition.

Tai Ji

There is one more mind-body tradition from Asia that has been repeatedly demonstrated to offer concurrent psychological and physical gains for neurological populations: Tai Ji (TJ, often written erroneously as Tai Chi), developed in China during the twelfth/thirteenth centuries CE, and is often credited as the creation of Daoist (Taoist) priests (see later), and subsequently spread to the wider Jinese populace and pioneered through unique styles linked to particular families (Yeates, 2015). TJ practice is characterised by slow, soft, flowing movements of all parts of the body, alongside breath regulation and deep psychological immersion in the movements. It is practiced as both a martial art (and is indeed the world's most popular martial art) and health cultivation practice. TJ forms the main focus of this chapter going forward, but here I introduce the main findings from the rapidly growing clinical evidence base of the use of TJ with different neurological populations. In subsequent sections of this chapter, I explore the theological and psychological dimension of TJ practice, and how this may inform future use of TJ within neuro-rehabilitation.

The scientific study of TJ in the general population has demonstrated gains in physical, cognitive and emotional functioning plus biophysical structural differences for regular practitioners (Jahnke et al., 2012). A review of TJ group trials with long-term complex conditions concluded there was evidence of both physical and psychological gains of TJ practice within these groups (Zhang et al., 2011). The strongest and most established evidence base for the use of TJ with specific neurological conditions is with Parkinson's disease and stroke, and primarily evidence of gains in physical functioning from participation in TJ groups.

In the Parkinsons disease literature, large-sample group studies (Gao et al., 2014; Li et al., 2012) have demonstrated gains in balance, postural stability and differing aspects of mobility for TJ practitioners relative to control groups, validating similar findings in smaller-sample studies (Vergara-Diaz et al., 2018; Hackney & Earhart, 2008). These findings are consistent with conclusions drawn from broader reviews of both English- and Chinese- literature studies (Mazzarin et al., 2017; Ni, Liu, Lu, Shi, & Guo, 2014; Toh, 2013; Radder et al., 2017; Yang, Li, Gong, Zhu, & Hao, 2014; Zhou et al., 2015).

A lower incidence of falls was reported in a post-TJ intervention follow-up period by Gao and colleagues (2014), compared with controls. A systematic review and meta-analysis by Winser, Tsang, Krishnamurthy, and Kannan (2018) concluded that there is strong evidence for improvement in balance and reduction in falls in people with either Parkinson's or stroke, with weaker evidence for this outcome in other conditions.

With regards to reviews of the stroke rehabilitation literature, Lyu and colleagues (2018) found TJ to have an overall beneficial effect on activities of daily living, balance, limb motor function, walking quality, mood and sleep from low-quality, evidence-based studies. Zheng, Zhou, Xia, Tao, and Chen (2016) found that when compared with standard physically orientated rehabilitation, TJ conferred significant gains in the areas of balance function, gait speed, anxiety and quality of life, in their meta-analysis of 15 eligible studies from both the English and Chinese language scientific literature. In contrast, no advantages were evident for survivor levels of depression or functional walking quality. Ding (2012) concluded from a review of five studies that TJ confers advantageous gains to stroke survivors in the domains of balance, mobility, quality of life, anxiety and depression. Gains in balance is the most replicated outcome across studies, concluded in reviews by Wu and colleagues (2018), Yan Li, Wang, Liu, and Zhang (2018) and Zou, Wang, Chen, and Wang (2018). Similar practices, such as baduanjin qi gong, have also been shown across studies to improve balance and other aspects of physical functioning, while reducing levels of depression, among other indices (Zou et al., 2018).

In terms of specific studies, a large-sample (n = 244) study by Xie and colleagues (2018) identified gains in motor functioning, fear of falling and depression when compared with a balance training control intervention. Taylor-Piliae and colleagues (2014) found Yang-style TJ for an older stroke survivors (>50) group to have had fewer falls than aerobic and treatment as usual control groups. Both TJ and aerobic control conferred better aerobic endurance than treatment as usual. No group effect was found for perceived mental health – all groups reported this. Wang and colleagues (2010) found positive differences for a TJ stroke group on measures of sleep quality/daytime dysfunction (including fatigue) and depressive symptoms. TJ interventions have been shown to improve standing balance in an older-adults sample (Au-Yeung, Hui-Chan, & Tang, 2009), and a sample of community-based stroke survivors reported gains in both general functioning and mood, alongside no adverse effects for practitioners (Hart et al., 2004). Hwang and colleagues (2017) found that an adapted TJ group for stroke survivors with hemiplegia that lasted for one year (10 participants completed all sessions) was characterized by improvements in balance, self-efficacy and flexibility on quantitative measures, alongside identification within qualitative interviews highlighting positive improvements for participants in physical and psychological functioning, social support and activities of daily living. A qualitative analysis of stroke survivor experiences in a TJ group by Desrochers, Kairy, Pan, Corriveau, and Tousignant (2016) highlighted simultaneous perceived physical and psychological benefits by participants. Interestingly, TJ has been applied to intentionally reduce risk factors to prevent the incidence of stroke in those who are at risk (Chan, Sit, & Chair, 2017).

Another key subgroup of acquired brain injury, traumatic brain injury (TBI) has been investigated in TJ studies, but using much smaller samples. Gemmell and Leathem (2006) have studied the psychosocial benefits for nine TBI survivors from a brief (six weeks) TJ group intervention, and reported participants' improved levels of sadness, confusion, anger, tension, fear and increased energy on visual analogue scales. Blake and Batson (2006) used a randomised design to demonstrate improvements in mood and self-esteem but not physical functioning in a TJ versus control group (20 participants in each condition). The authors concluded that their results were inconclusive as a recommendation for the use of TJ with TBI survivors. A similarly powered study by Mańko, Ziółkowski, Mirski, and Kłosiński (2013) found modest evidence for self-care gains unique to a six-weeks rehabilitation programme incorporating TJ exercises when compared with a standard rehabilitation intervention for survivors of severe TBI who had been in prolonged comas. Finally, Shapira, Chelouche, Yanai, Kaner, and Szold (2001) report three case studies where TBI survivors who had participated in TJ reported gains in mobility and feelings of security while walking.

Other neurological conditions have also been studied in the TJ literature. A systematic review of studies investigating TJ for people with multiple sclerosis concluded that it is safe and confers both physical and psychological benefits (Taylor & Taylor-Piliae, 2017). In a twice-weekly TJ group for people with multiple sclerosis, Burschka, Keune, Oy, Oschman, and Kuhn (2014) found a small effect size (sample of 32 participants) for therapeutic gains in balance, coordination, and levels of depression relative to a treatment as usual group. Tavee, Rensel, Planchon, Butler, and Stone (2011) found improvements in ratings of pain, and physical and mental health functioning in a two-month TJ group for people with multiple sclerosis (n=22) relative to a control intervention. These findings are consistent with those reported by smaller sample studies conducted by Mills and Allen (2000).

Gains from TJ have also been reported for people with mild cognitive impairment (reduction of falls, Sungkarat et al., 2017) and cerebellar ataxia (balance and functional independence, Winser, Kannan, Pang, & Tsang, 2017; Winser et al.,

2018). Finally, Quinn and Jones (2012) reported a range of psychosocial gains following completion of a TJ group for people with a variety of neurological conditions. Yeates and colleagues (submitted; Yeates in press a, in press b) also report positive single-case outcomes for a small group of survivors of ABI following a six-month TJ group but also draw attention to significant diversity in this group and the influence of such on the range of outcomes within the group

In summary, the existing literature points reliably to a range of physical functioning gains across neurological conditions, although the evidence is strongest and most reliable in Parkinson's disease and stroke. Conclusions for other conditions are limited by small sample sizes and differing outcome measures. There are two key problems with this literature as a whole, however. A general critique is that the most rigorously designed studies have optimised participant homogeneity by excluding those participants with significant cognitive difficulties alongside their physical impairments (e.g., Taylor-Piliae et al., 2014). This then creates a barrier to applying the findings of these studies to the users of services described earlier in this chapter, who are struggling with multiple domains of disability (Yeates, 2015, 2018, in press a, in press b; Yeates et al., submitted). More recently, Hwang and colleagues (2017) have been the first to describe physical adaptations to a TJ group for stroke survivors with hemiplegia.

Furthermore, most studies have operationalised physical functioning measures as the primary outcome only. Where psychological functioning has been additionally studied, it is clear from the foregoing findings that reduction in anxiety and depression is often found by investigators. However, these have not been the main focus of each study, nor have investigators offered explanatory frameworks to explain the link between performing TJ movements and emotional wellbeing. Burschka and colleagues (2014) did offer mindfulness as a possible explanatory framework for these empirical associations, but as we explore later, this is not the key mind-body framework that TJ experts use themselves to guide their practice.

Mind-body approaches with aphasia

The mind-body approaches reviewed earlier may offer a unique form of support for people with communication problems. It is clear that mindfulness, yoga and TJ are both physical and talking therapies, the focus on the body in these approaches predominates over a verbal exchange as the supportive mechanism. Verbal comprehension of the body work and the intended aims for mental wellbeing is a requirement, but is augmented by the visual observational and embodied learning that characterise these practices. Where comprehension is unaffected, expressive difficulties present fewer participation barriers in and psychological gains to practitioners with a range of neurological conditions in contrast to talking psychological interventions.

To date, few studies have explicitly reported on the use of mind-body interventions for people with aphasia. In fact, the presence of aphasia is a common exclusion criterion for those investigators seeking homogenous samples (see earlier and Yeates, 2015, 2018). Existing studies have reported the use of such interventions with participants with primarily expressive aphasia.

Yoga is one mind-body practice where clinicians are developing specific adaptations to maximise involvement of people with aphasia (Ross, Howe, Jenstad, & Sinden, 2018), although aside from a case study that reports mixed findings (Rivkin, unpublished thesis), an evaluation of these approaches remains outstanding. Several case study reports of mindfulness meditation as applied following aphasia are published. The impact of this approach on divided attention in people with aphasia has been investigated by Orenstein, Basilakos, and Shisler Marshall (2012), and Laures-Gore and Marshall (2016) reported improvements on both psychophysiological (heart rate, heart-rate variability), cognitive (decreased impulsivity, improved attention) and communication performance (word production, phrase length, word generation) measures in an individual with aphasia (14 years post stroke) following a five-day mindfulness meditation training. This group extended their approach to a small group study, finding a superior but non-significant difference in the five-day mindfulness training group versus controls (Shisler-Marshall, Lores-Gore, & Love, 2017). In a post-stroke aphasia case study reported by Dickenson and colleagues (2016), significant reductions in anxiety alongside communication gains (improvements in confrontation naming picture description and repetition) were reported. The authors made the case that approaches such as mindfulness meditation may offer a way to break the disabling negative interactions between anxiety and exacerbation of communication restrictions in people with aphasia. Finally, Crielesi and colleagues (this volume) reported both single-case study material and data from a small group evaluation of a mindfulness group to highlight gains in psychological functioning and quality of life indicators. While embryonic in nature, this collection of studies tentatively highlights the potential of mind-body practices to offer gains across multiple domains of functioning in people with aphasia.

Daoist frameworks for Tai Ji, qi gong and Flow-based practices

The omissions in the scientific literature described previously are all the more significant when one considers that those expert TJ practitioners who practice the most, for the longest and prioritise this practice above other aspects of life, all hold the internal, subjective (psychological) dimension to be central to their practice. *Taijiquan* means the representation of the universe (in the Daoist view) through bodily movement. It is still practiced by the Daoist monastic community to this day, as well as having millions of other practitioners worldwide, of all ages, backgrounds and abilities. For the Daoist monk TJ masters, despite their mastery and prowess of physical movements, balance and coordination, their focus is on their internal experience in harmony with both their bodily movements and wider universal natural processes, all connected within their view of natural laws and organisation. This is a unique bio-psycho-social-spiritual-ecological framework, which is explored here.

Daoism is a key indigenous religion of China. Practiced by at least 20 million people in China and worldwide, Daoism was formalised in the second century CE but is thought to have developed from preceding shamanic beliefs and co-developed in reciprocal dialogue with Chan Buddhism and Confucionism, the other two main spiritual-philosophical traditions in pre-communist China. The Daoist view of the divine is an emanating universal force that proceeds and evolves, underlying all the manifestations of change and transition in the natural world and wider universe. This process is called *Dao*, which translates as the 'way' or 'path'. Nature is a key source of inspiration to connect with the divine in Daoism, through witnessing and harmonising one's lifestyle with changing seasons, differing states and qualities of essential elements such as water (ice, fog, mist, rivers and lakes). This harmonisation of lifestyle is done via horticultural practices, herbology, musical and architectural styles and mind-body practices. The body is viewed as a manifestation of nature and subject to its laws (yin – receiving, embracing, yielding forces, and yang – emanating, protruding, opening forces). As such, one's body, and the interrelationship between the body and the embodied mind (see later) is seen as a domain in which a Daoist can intentionally promote harmony with nature.

This harmonisation and health cultivation process in the level of body, mind and spirit is referred to as 'Neidan', or 'Inner Alchemy'. The practitioner aims to self-harmonise with natural processes and facilitate a key process of conversion – from their bodily essence/physical properties ('Jing') their physical attributes are used in service of breath regulation to stimulate and circulate a Flow of vitality and life energy ('Qi') around the body. This circulation alters the mind and subjective experience of the practitioner, leading to expanded States of consciousness. These final processes are conceived as the domain of spirit ('Shen'), but different qualities of mind-spirit are anchored to specific mind-body physiological networks, with links to specific organs (including the heart, lungs, kidneys and liver). This echoes more contemporary developments in neuroscience that highlight interoceptive processes mediated by subcortical-viscera networks that are generative of consciousness (Damasio, 1999). This conversion of body-breath/life energy-spirit is completed by the highest converted essence being put back into the universe. As such, the body, breath, mind and spirit are all vehicles and containers for a never-ending Flow of universal change processes that permeate all things. The aim then, is to minimise blocks and desynchronies that would obstruct this process.

The Neidan process is a core focus of seated Daoist meditational practices but is also the organiser for a range of mind-body practices such as TJ, qi gong (still or moving yogic practices that typically involve greater repetition of fewer movements than TJ), and gong fu (kung fu – faster and more dynamic practices with a clear martial focus). Furthermore, music, chanting of hymns and scriptures, horticulture, cooking and eating, architecture, divination and sleeping are also used as lifestyle vehicles for Neidan to aim towards a constant trend towards harmonisation with nature and the divine.

Poetry and literature are also key mediums for the Daoist philosophical exploration of divine change, famously including the *Dao De Ching*, attributed in Chinese folklore to a semi-historical/mythological figure, Lao Tzu (Kaltenmark, 1969). In ancient Daoist writings, philosophical ideas were communicated powerfully through imagery and allegory, famously including Zhuangzi's (fourth-century BC) Butterfly Dream:

> Once upon a time, I, Chuang Chou, dreamt I was a butterfly, fluttering hither and thither, to all intents and purposes a butterfly. I was conscious only of my happiness as a butterfly, unaware that I was Chou. Soon I awoke, and there I was, veritably myself again. Now I do not know whether I was then a man dreaming I was a butterfly, or whether I am now a butterfly, dreaming I am a man. Between a man and a butterfly there is necessarily a distinction. The transition is called the transformation of material things.
>
> (cited in Merton, 1969)

In Daoist practice, these ideas of mind-body work and harmonisation with change are then located within a broader environmental context, the surrounding natural world and universe. Five Element Theory ('Wuxing') is a framework that is constantly used to link parts of the body, emotions, the changing seasonal environment and diet to promote synchronisation. For example, I am writing this chapter in autumn, where the leaves falling from the bare trees remind the Chinese of the structure of a lung, so body movements are chosen to stimulate respiration, along with the increased consumption of spices. The key element is metal, consistent with the sensory properties of lung tissue and the smell of decaying leaf matter in the ground. The prominent emotion and subjective State is sorrow and sadness, with nature providing lessons of loss and exposed vulnerability.

Nature provides inspiration for a model of mind, behaviour and interaction with others. For example, the bending of the willow under the weight of snowfall is contrasted with a rigid tree such as a fir that seems stronger on the surface, but in its rigidity does not yield and so breaks under the weight of the snow. Thus, the concept of 'Wu Wei' is a guiding principal – a Daoist tries to respond to external stimulation and challenge through initially yielding and accommodating – not jumping forwards with judgements, preconceptions and bulldozing into situations. The sage or hermit in harmony with nature and not overly organised by societal expectations is a key archetypal template for Daoist psychological and social life. TJ is practiced within this biopsychosocial-spiritual-ecological framework. Given this brief overview of the Daoist view of the embodied mind and spirit within the cosmos, the physiological reductionism of TJ research becomes stark.

Flow psychology

Therefore, in contrast to TJ as a physical practice only, we have a rich range of Daoist concepts that both guide internal experience during bodily practice and situate such within a wider ecological and lifestyle context. One limitation is that these concepts are esoteric and not easily accessible. These core concepts do, however, overlap significantly with some key ideas within Western positive psychology, a broad contemporary influence on neuro-rehabilitation (Cullen et al., 2018; Evans, 2011; Evans & Cullen, in press). Mihály Csíkszentmihályi (1990, 1997) has developed the concept of Flow, a concept which can potentially offer an explanatory bridge between Daoist terminology and scientific-clinical discourse (Yeates, 2015, 2018). Indeed, Csíkszentmihályi (1990) has explicitly identified another Eastern mind-body tradition, yoga, as a purposefully designed Flow activity:

> The similarities between Yoga and Flow are extremely strong; in fact it makes sense to think that (Patanjali's system of) Yoga is a very thoroughly planned Flow activity'; p 105, 'Therefore it is not unreasonable to view Yoga as one of the oldest and most systematic methods of producing the Flow experience.
> (p. 105)

Csíkszentmihályi has primarily studied intense States of absorption in the domains of sport, music, creativity and work. Flow States are routinely described by practitioners as involving the dissolving of a self-State and loss of normal self-boundaries (loss of reflective self-consciousness), distortion of temporal experience, a merging of action and awareness where intention is not effortful and the activity concerned seems to Flow forth of its own accord. Practitioners feel intense wellbeing, ecstatic experiences at the time and part of something bigger than themselves. Importantly, those experiencing Flow States in a particular activity have attained some level of mastery over that activity through practice and experience, such that there is a dimension of automaticity and diminution of effort. Practitioners across diverse fields consistently use a metaphorical language of creativity and action Flowing forth, hence Csíkszentmihályi's term 'Flow States'. Many of us know what it is to be 'in the Flow', and the value of such, when we think about optimal times for our own performance and productivity. Flow has been associated with optimal psychological wellbeing (Csíkszentmihályi, 1990, 1997), and a specific focus on Flow has been included in a positive psychotherapy intervention that was shown to be acceptable for survivors of ABI, with a recommendation for a future trial of this approach in ABI (Cullen et al., 2018).

Csíkszentmihályi acknowledged historical precursors to his psychological study of Flow, notably religious thought from near and far Eastern traditions. Many faiths have historically articulated and practiced a desired goal to be at oneness with something greater, via dissolution of the boundaries of present sensory experience. In addition to Daoism, these include in Islam, Sufi Dervishes' practice of spinning and whirling; in Vedic/Hindu thought, a form of Flow-like psychological absorption in an object of meditation, Samyama, aimed for in Raja Yoga and fast forms of physical Yoga Flow States are explicitly the desired vehicles for self-transcendence; Gregorian chanting in Christianity and the use of prayer beads and repetition of prayer forms/mantras in all the major faiths.

The concept of Flow is explicitly mentioned by exponents of the Daoist worldview, famously Bruce Lee:

> Be like water . . . empty your mind, be formless, shapeless like water. If you put water in the cup, it becomes the cup. You put water in the bottle, it becomes the bottle. You put it in the teapot, it becomes the teapot. Now, water can Flow or it can crash. Be water, my friend.
>
> (Little & Lee, 2000, TV documentary)

> We are always in a process of becoming, and nothing is fixed. Have no rigid system in you, and you'll be flexible to change with the ever changing. Open yourself and Flow, my friend. Flow in the total openness of the living moment. If nothing within you stays rigid, outward things will disclose themselves. Moving, be like water. Still, be like a mirror. Respond like an echo.
>
> (2000, p. 13)

While there is clearly overlap between Daoist and positive psychological conceptualisation of Flow States, the latter differs in emphasising explicit appraisal as a critical dimension. This includes assertions of Flow components and conditions for Flow such as an individual's sense of personal control or agency, involvement in a task with a clear set of goals and progress, and which provides immediate feedback, simultaneous perception of high task challenges alongside high personal skill (Csíkszentmihályi, Abuhamdeh, & Nakamura, 2005; Schaffer, 2013). While Daoist masters clearly have mastery of highly skilled practices such as martial arts, accounts of their subjective experiences during practice indicate a diminution of explicit appraisal processes generally and subjective absence of perceived challenge or personal skill (see *The Taijiquan Classics*, Davis, 2004). Furthermore, the psychological study of people in Flow States has focused on those who have specific goals around performance (be this athletic or work productivity), with Flow States being a dimension towards these outcomes. The Daoist TJ masters aspire specifically to enter into Flow States and the opportunities for transcendence and wider harmony, irrespective of their performance (although it is clear that their physical and psychological abilities exceed most in the general population).

Liminality and psychological growth

With change and transformation processes afforded such psychological and spiritual significance, the dimension of change is seen as the domain in which personal development occurs. This is commensurate with the focus across cultures and human experience on *liminality*, which has become an area of transdisciplinary academic and applied clinical interest. Liminal experiences are seen as self-experience within a phase of transition (between what someone once was and what they are becoming) and being of psychological value. Anthropologists have noted the centrality of liminal experience in rites of passage across cultures, where this phase (such as adolescent transition between childhood and adulthood) is marked by ceremony and symbolism. Narratives of passing through gates and portals permeate all of the major religions, be these processes of change in behaviour and learning or the unlocking of centres within the body. Psychotherapy too has been conceived as an arena where:

> a new set of circumstances involve the dissolution of a former identity and the formation of a new identity. Between these two States, the condition of liminality suspends a person or system in what may appear to be an amorphous or ill-defined State.
>
> (Elliot, 2011)

Growth and adaptation are viewed as emergent from such conditions. To link back to the experiences of ABI survivors, adjustment, awareness and post-injury growth can be limited by a rigid investment in pre-injury identity in a way that devalues post-injury change and closes down growth opportunities (Tyerman & Humphrey, 1984). A Daoist-focused exploration of the course of change itself rather than the privileging of one particular State in that journey may create new rehabilitation opportunities. An example would be comparing the relative attributes and limitations of different values and abilities at different points in time, in response to varying life conditions and demands post injury.

Using Flow states to guide Tai Ji groups in neuro-rehabilitation

The extrapolation of concepts from Daoist psychology, by way of a translation with the Western concept of Flow, has provided us with a new psychological tool to be used in clinical application. Because there was once a time before people were using the mindfulness concept across a range of sectors, the concept of Flow awaits a future explosion of clinical application. It is argued here (and in Yeates, 2015, 2018), that Flow provides the core operationalisation of a psychological (and for some a spiritual) dimension in the formulation and implementation of TJ groups for people with neuro-disability. Flow is significant for TJ clinical interventions in two main ways – firstly, it links the bodily movements with the evidenced psychological gains from TJ practice, commensurate with positive psychology's identification of psychological wellbeing correlates with Flow States. This may offer a unique response to the existential disturbances to self-experience described earlier. To use the Daoist inspirations from the natural world, think of leaves floating in a stream. They are individual elements, but when moved simultaneously in the Flow of currents and eddies in the stream, they are held in unison by a higher level of process or organisation. Similarly, survivors of ABI, initially experiencing themselves as fragmented, 'in pieces', can be temporarily held together by the TJ movement sequence, also perhaps held together by moving in unison with fellow TJ practitioners (akin to a murmuration of starlings or a shoal of fish), and for some there may be an experience of synchrony and union with a higher principle – a transcendent experience.

Secondly, it can provide the specificity to optimise Flow experience (with associated conditions of improved psychological wellbeing and the possibility of transcendence) for each practitioner in a bespoke fashion. If Flow emerges from the optimal ratio of perceived challenge and ability to meet that challenge, then specific movements are chosen that fit this ratio for each survivor (with their unique constellation of physical, cognitive, emotional and social needs). Furthermore, specific compensatory rehabilitation strategies are included as adjuncts to optimise the learning and practice of TJ (see Table 8.1 for examples), again to promote and optimise Flow.

Table 8.1 Examples of adaptations to Tai Ji learning and practice for different post-stroke difficulties

Area of difficulty	*Suggested adaptation*
Mobility	Chair-based sequences and/or restricted standing TJ forms.
Balance	Chair-based sequences, and/or TJ forms that have minimal weight and direction changes.
Hemiplegia	Use of therapy bands, sticks and bilateral hand connection to mobilise mirroring upper-body movements, visual imagery of paralysed limb movement; focus on trunk movement to amplify functional movement of ipsilateral limbs.
Fatigue	Do short sequences of instruction and movement, slowly increasing over time. Regular breaks.
Dyspraxia	Use tactile feedback and physical adjustments rather than relying on visual demonstration alone.
Communication	Emphasis on visual and kinaesthetic teaching as opposed to verbal-based teaching.
Attention	Do short sequences of instruction and movement, slowly increasing over time. Regular breaks. Use of key phrases and words for optimal alerting qualities.
Episodic memory/new learning	Focus on errorless learning in class to minimise the introduction of mistakes into the learning process. For those who want to learn sequences at home, use of DVDs/internet videos to provide a guide between session times and promote a greater number of repetition learning experiences. Also supporting the autonomous learning of a sequence through backward-chaining rather than traditional instruction.
Topographical disorientation/ visuo-spatial difficulties in using allocentric or egocentric cues	Use grids marked on the floor to assist with changing directions of movement and posture shapes.

Area of difficulty	*Suggested adaptation*
Anxiety	Use of relaxing music, short teaching sequences. Teaching of body-tension reduction and breath-regulation strategies at the beginning of the class. Reducing the learning/practice demands of the movements initially to increase confidence, then gently introducing progressively more challenging sequences.
Low mood	Shorter learning/practice phases; pacing the progressive challenge of sequences as described earlier, supporting achievements with praise and encouragement, emphasising the group fellowship and identity aspects of attendance. Drawing comparison to embodied experience at the end of the session versus the beginning.

The systematic use of Flow in this way to optimise psychological wellbeing within TJ practice for survivors of ABI and people with other forms of disability would result in two different practitioners performing very different movement sequences (each with varying physical and psychological demands) and using very different compensatory strategies, but both entering into a similar State of Flow within their practice (having arrived at it, entered into it, through different routes). Within a TJ group intervention (a Flow Group, © Yeates 2016), the session would be structured to offer both time devoted to individual learning of bespoke movements and also an additional segment of group movement sequences (accessible to all attendees) to facilitate the experience of group cohesion with others, plus a dedicated time for socialising and peer connection during a tea break.

With regards to people with aphasia specifically, Sather (2015) has highlighted both the capacity of this population to access Flow State experience, but also the powerful role of environmental (physical environment and other people) and personal factors to act as supports or barriers to Flow experience. To provide more details on the value of TJ and the experience of Flow for a survivor of ABI struggling with expressive aphasia, a case study is described next.

Case example: Andy

Andy, 44, sustained a left middle cerebral artery infarction six years previously, which involved the left posterior frontal and anterior parietal lobes, including Broca's area. In addition to expressive aphasia (but relatively intact comprehension) and right hemiparesis affecting his lower and upper limbs, enduring cognitive difficulties evident in neuropsychological assessment six years post injury included impairments in attention, memory and the formation of plans in response to problems/goals. Andy's mood was low; he was dependent on cannabis to manage these feelings plus anxiety when anticipating dealing/communicating with others. He was socially isolated. Andy had attempted to return to work in a supermarket post stroke, but this had not been successful and had eroded his confidence even further. His experiences in accessing psychological support were mostly negative and included both a lack of referrals to talking therapies and one experience of becoming frustrated during a counselling session when he was unable to adequately convey his experiences.

He engaged with the author's community service to primarily receive vocational support, and he declined the offer of talking psychological therapy, given his previous experiences. A pilot study of a six-month TJ group was being conducted in this service, and this was offered to Andy. He was very interested and accepted readily – the idea of a bodily-based activity to relax and be with other people, moving quietly without the need to make much conversation, really appealed. It was a unique opportunity in a world that is so focused on verbal conversational exchange.

As part of the research project, he completed questionnaires measuring anxiety and depression (Hospital Anxiety & Depression Scale, HADS, Zigmond & Snaith, 1983), and fatigue (Modified Fatigue Impact Scale, M-FIS, Fisk et al., 1994) on a repeating basis every four weeks. In addition, Andy completed a Quality of Life (Quality of Life after Brain Injury Inventory, QOLiBRI, ref) questionnaire before the first session and following the last session of the intervention. Clinical significance of changes in scores were determined using severity categories and cut-offs published for each scale, where the statistical reliability of score changes was evaluated using the Reliable Change Index (Jacobson & Truax, 1991).

Andy attended 88% of the six-month, weekly sessions. His scores on these measures before and after the six-month TJ group are reported in Table 8.2.

Andy's scores on these measures across the four-week repeated measures data collection schedule are graphed in Figures 8.1 and 8.2.

Andy's levels of anxiety and fatigue remained constant during the six months, while his levels of depressive symptomatology significantly and reliably decreased

Table 8.2 Andy's mood, fatigue and quality of life data

Measure	*Pre-TJ*	*Post-TJ*	*Significance?*
HADS anxiety	9	9	Mild, no change
HADS depression	11	6	Moderate to normal range, reliable
MFIS total	60	51	Modest reduction in fatigue, not reliable
MFIS physical subscale	35	30	n/a
MFIS cognitive subscale	17	19	n/a
MFIS psychosocial	8	2	n/a
QoLiBRI total	29	44	No change

Note: HADS = Hospital Anxiety & Depression Scale; MFIS = Modified Fatigue Impact Scale; QoLIBRI = Quality of Life in Brain Injury Scale

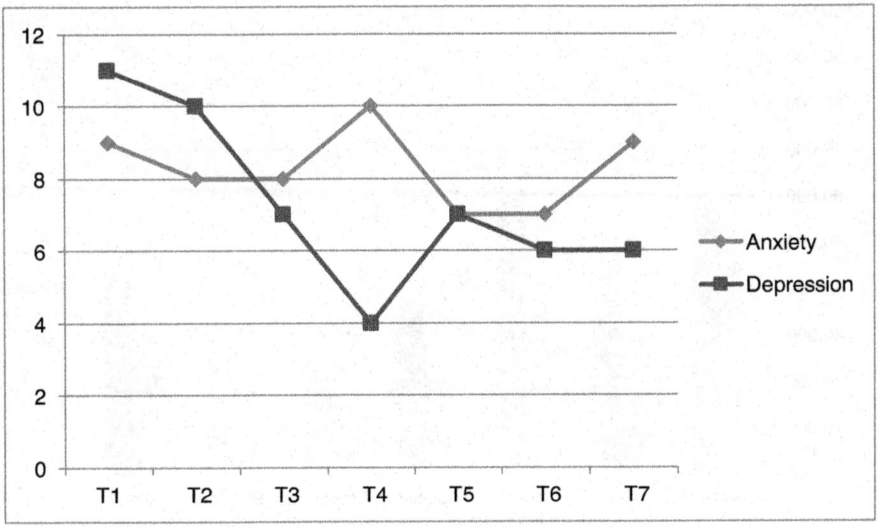

Figure 8.1 Andy's anxiety and depression (HADS) scores across sessions during the six-month Tai Ji group

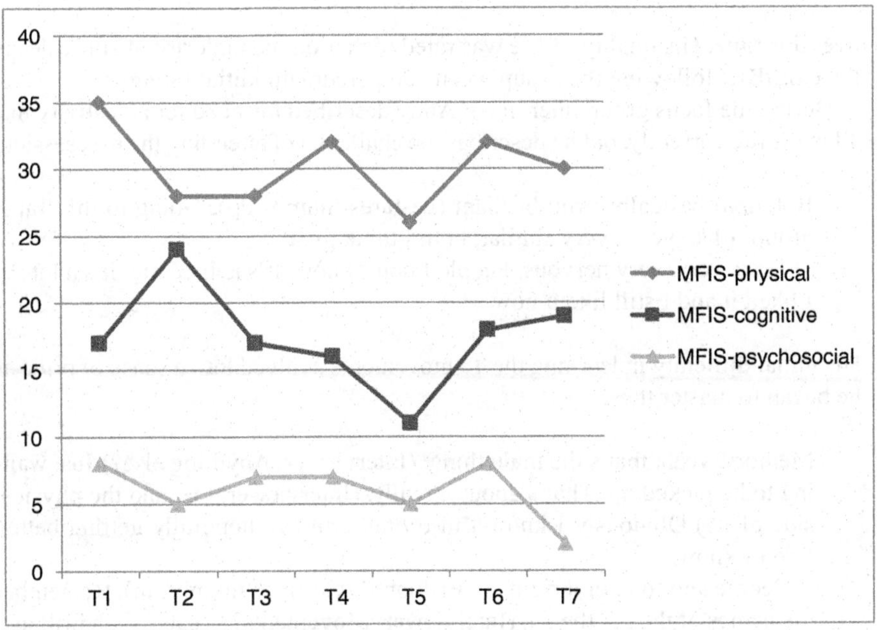

Figure 8.2 Andy's fatigue (MFIS) scores across sessions during the six-month Tai Ji group

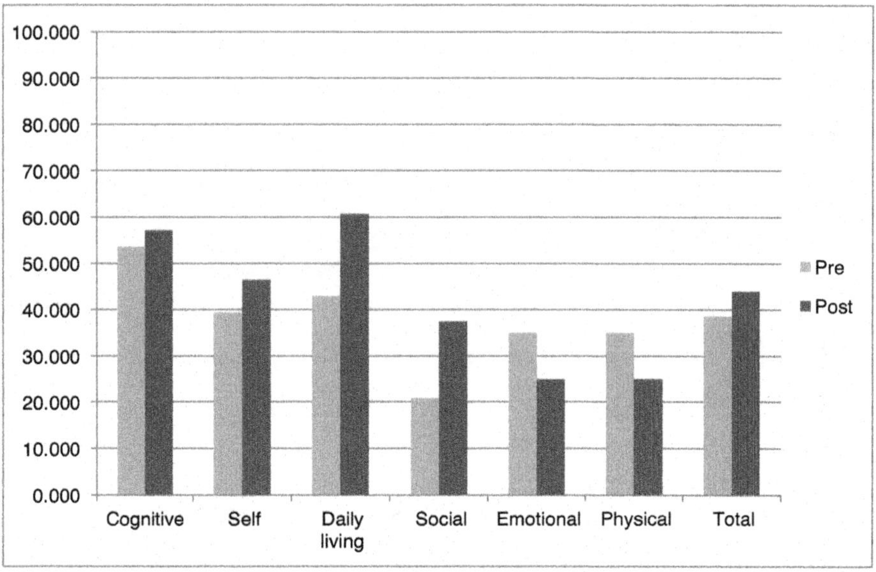

Figure 8.3 Andy's quality of life (QoLIBRI subscales) scores before and after the six-month Tai Ji group

over this time. His quality of life was rated higher on the majority of subscales in the QoLiBRI following the group when compared with initial ratings.

During the focus group interviews, Andy described his need for an activity like TJ in his life currently, but he describes the challenge of attending the first session:

> Boredom basically, erm, brilliant (gestures thumbs up). Going to this Tai Ji group. I like yoga, very similar, both I think great.
>
> I was very, very nervous. People I don't know. It's helped me, it's a lot . . . I liked it and I still like it now.

His initial difficulty in learning the TJ movements evolved into a sense of pride as he began to master these:

> Memory, yeah, that's the main thing. (Interviewer: Anything else?) Just waiting to be picked up. That's about it really. (Interviewer: OK and the physical side of it?) Obviously I know I'm trying, erm . . . hopefully getting better, I don't know.
>
> People and 'oh got it right . . . Brilliant!' (Gestures thumbs up). Remember the names of the . . . the . . . (Interviewer: Movements?) Yeah . . . oh brilliant. I've done it. (Interviewer: Like a sense of achievement, you've done it?) Yeah, yeah . . . I remember the moves, I . . . every two days I . . . (Interviewer: Practice at home?) Yeah, yeah.

In the final focus group at the end of the six-month TJ programme, Andy described the key benefits, despite the physical challenges:

> Well, sometimes it's a bit hard for me anyway . . . with one hand (Interviewer: Physically) . . . yeah . . . I like to go and practice obviously and get better . . . yeah calmer . . . every day . . . just relaxing muscles and every day now I just relaxing and calmer.

INTERVIEWER: So this is an activity for you? And for the social aspect of it?
ANDY: Exactly! Yes, yeah, yeah.

In summary, the TJ group was hugely significant in Andy's life in reducing his depression and offering a social, leisure and activity opportunity that was not dependent on verbal communication. His diligence in practicing the movements at home was a key indicator of engagement in the programme. He valued being in a community of Tai Ji practitioners, his training partners, while not facing the frequent challenges and anxieties associated with verbal communication that plagued the majority of his life since the stroke. His embodied practice of the TJ forms and sequences, and inclusion in a group activity that is not defined by language expression competence, all was characterised by Flow. For Andy, Flow was typically absent in other aspects of his life, as a socially excluded person with aphasia and other cognitive, physical and emotional challenges, jarring and out of synch with the people and lifestyles around him. The measured changes in aspects of his mental health and psychological wellbeing as concomitants of these Flow experiences demonstrate the value of these opportunities for Andy and other people with aphasia.

Conclusions and future directions

The role of Eastern mind-body practices (with a key focus on Tai Ji) in promoting the psychological wellbeing of people with aphasia following different forms of acquired brain injury has been presented, via a literature review, conceptual exploration from both clinical and Eastern spiritual literatures, and finally an illustrative case study. Given the verbal focus of most forms of psychological support (and the demonstrated excluding outcomes for people with aphasia as a result), the valued contribution of embodied practices such as Tai Ji require further exploration. Systematic evaluation is required of TJ groups focused specifically on people with aphasia, to parallel the current embryonic developments in yoga within stroke services. The foregoing case study illustrated the beneficial impact of a TJ group that was not specifically adapted in terms of the delivery and support of TJ practice for people with aphasia, but it is likely that greater gains could be achieved if communication adaptations such as those reported earlier were key elements of future intervention protocols. In any case, the use of mind-body practices such as Tai Ji represent a long-awaited paradigm shift away from verbal primacy in the emotional support of people with aphasia.

Note

1 Consultant clinical neuropsychologist and Wudang Tai Ji/Kung Fu instructor

References

Advocat, J., Enticott, J., Vandenberg, B., Hassed, C., Hester, J., & Russell, G. (2016). The effects of a mindfulness-based lifestyle program for adults with Parkinson's disease: A mixed methods, wait list controlled randomised control study. *BMC Neurology*, *16*, 166.

Aghabagheri, H., Mohammadkhani, P., Omrani, S., & Farahmand, V. (2012). Mindfulness based group therapy on Increase in subjective well-being and hope to MS patients. *Clinical Psychology*, *4*(1), 23–23.

Au-Yeung, S. S. Y., Hui-Chan, C. W. Y., & Tang, J. C. S. (2009). Short-form Tai Chi improves standing balance of people with chronic stroke. *Neurorehabilitation & Neural Repair*, *23*, 515–522.

Baker, C., Worrall, R. M., Hudson, K., Ryan, B., & O'Byrne, L. (2018). A systematic review of rehabilitation interventions to prevent and treat depression in post-stroke aphasia. *Disability & Rehabilitation, 40*(16), 1870–1892.

Bastille, J. V., & Gill-Body, K. M. (2004). A yoga-based exercise program for people with post-stroke chronic hemiparesis. *Physical Therapy*, *84*, 33–48.

Bedard, M., Felteau, M., Gibbons, C., Klein, R., Mazmanian, D., Fedyk, K., & Mack, G. (2005). A mindfulness-based intervention to improve quality of life among individuals who sustained traumatic brain injuries: One-year follow-up. *The Journal of Cognitive Rehabilitation*, Spring, 2–7.

Bedard, M., Felteau, M., Marshall, S., Dubois, S., Gibbons, C., Klein, R., & Weaver, B. (2012). Mindfulness-based cognitive therapy: Benefits in reducing depression following a traumatic brain injury. *Advances in Mind-Body Medicine*, *26*, 14–20.

Bedard, M., Felteau, M., Mazmanian, D., Fedyk, K., Klein, R., Richardson, J. . . . Minthorn-Biggs, M. B. (2003). Pilot evaluation of a mindfulness-based intervention to improve quality of life among individuals who sustained traumatic brain injuries. *Disability and Rehabilitation*, *25*, 722–731.

Behn, N., Hilari, K., Marshall, J., Simpson, A., Northcott, S., & Thomas, S. (2018). Supporting well-being through PEeR-Befriending (SUPERB_ trial: An exploration of fidelity in peer-befriending for people with aphasia. *Aphasiology*, *32*(supp 1), 21–25.

Bishop, S. R., Shapiro, S., Carlson, L., Anderson, N. D., Carmody, J., Segal, Z. V. . . . Devins, G. (2004). Mindfulness: A proposed operational definition. *Clinical Psychology: Science & Practice*, *11*, 230–241.

Blake, H., & Batson, M. (2006). Exercise intervention in brain injury: A pilot randomized study of Tai Chi Qigong. *Clinical Rehabilitation*, *23*(7), 589–598.

Blankespoor, R. J., Schellekens, M. P. J., Vos, S. H., Speckens, A. E. M., & de Jong, B. A. (2017). The effectiveness of mindfulness-based stress reduction on psychological distress and cognitive functioning in patients with multiple sclerosis: A pilot study. *Mindfulness*, *8*(5), 1251–1258. https://doi.org/10.1007/s12671-017-0701-6.

Bogosian, A., Chadwick, P., Windgassen, S., Norton, S., McCrone, P., Mosweu, I. . . . Moss-Morris, R. (2015). Distress improves after mindfulness training for progressive MS: A pilot randomised trial. *Multiple Sclerosis Journal*, *21*(9), 1184–1194.

Bogosian, A., Hughes, A., Norton, S., Silber, E., & Moss-Morris, R. (2016). Potential treatment mechanisms in a mindfulness based intervention for people with progressive multiple sclerosis. *British Journal of Health Psychology*, *21*(4), 859–880.

Bowen, C., Yeates, G., & Palmer, S. (2010). *A relational approach to rehabilitation: Thinking about relationships after brain injury*. London: Karnac.

Burschka, J. M., Keune, P. M., Oy, U., Oschman, P., & Kuhn, P. (2014). Mindfulness-based interventions in multiple sclerosis: Beneficial effects of Tai Chi on balance, coordination, fatigue and depression. *BioMedCentral Neurology*, *14*(1), 165–174.

Cash, T., Ekouevi, V., Kilbourn, C., & Lageman, S. (2015). Pilot study of a mindfulness-based group intervention for individuals with Parkinson's disease and their caregivers. *Mindfulness*, *7*(2), 361–371.

Chan, A. W., Sit, J. W., & Chair, S. Y. (2017). Tai Chi exercise reduces stroke risk factors: A randomized controlled trial. *Stroke*, *48*, AWP416.

Cramer, H., Lauche, R., Azizi, H., Dobos, G., & Langhorst, J. (2014). Yoga for multiple sclerosis: A systematic review and meta-analysis. *PLoS ONE*, *9*, e112414.

Crielesi, M., Monopoli, G., Yeates, G. N., & Monte, S. (In Press). A mindfulness group intervention for people with aphasia: A pilot study. In G. N. Yeates & K. Meredith (Eds.), *Neuro-disability & psychotherapy, specialist topics (Vol. II): Psychotherapy & aphasia: Supporting emotions & relationships*. Oxford: Routledge.

Cruice, M., Hill, R., Worrall, L., & Hickson, L. (2010). Conceptualizing quality of life in older people with aphasia. *Aphasiology*, *24*, 327–347.

Csíkszentmihályi, M. (1990). *Flow: The psychology of optimal experience*. New York: Harper & Row.

Csíkszentmihályi, M. (1997). *Finding flow: The psychology of engagement with everyday life*. New York: Basic Books.

Csíkszentmihályi, M., Abuhamdeh, S., & Nakamura, J. (2005). Flow. In A. Elliot (Ed.), *Handbook of competence and motivation* (pp. 598–698). New York: The Guilford Press.

Cullen, B., Pownall, J., Cummings, J., Baylan, S., Broomfield, N., Haig, C. . . . Evans, J. (2018). Positive PsychoTherapy in ABI rehab (PoPsTAR): A pilot randomised controlled trial. *Neuropsychological Rehabilitation*, *28*(1), 17–33.

Dalemans, R. J. P., Wade, D., Van den Heuvel, W., & De Witte, L. (2009). Facilitating the participation of people with aphasia in research: A description of strategies. *Clinical Rehabilitation*, *23*, 948–959.

Damasio, A. (1999). *The feeling of what happens*. San Diego, CA: Harcourt.

Davis, B. (2004). *The taijiquan classics: An annotated translation*. Berkeley, CA: North Atlantic.

Desrochers, P., Kairy, D., Pan, S., Corriveau, H., & Tousignant, M. (2016). Tai chi for upper limb rehabilitation in stroke patients: The patient's perspective. *Disability & Rehabilitation*, *39*(13), 1313–1319.

Detert, N., & Douglas, L. (2014). Mindfulness MBSR/MBCT improves general psychiatric symptom severity, depression, anxiety and perceived stress in neurological disorders in an NHS clinical setting. *Neuro-Disability & Psychotherapy*, *2*(1/2), 137–156.

Detert, V. (In Press). Mindfulness in neurological conditions. In G. N. Yeates & F. Ashworth (Eds.), *Psychological therapies in neuropsychological rehabilitation*. Hove: Psychology Press.

Ding, M. (2012). Tai Chi for stroke rehabilitation: A focused review. *American Journal of Physical Medicine & Rehabilitation*, *91*, 1091–1096. https://doi.org/10.1097/PHM.0b013e31826edd21

Dissanayaka, N. N., Idu Jion, F., Pachana, N. A., O'Sullivan, J. D., Marsh, R., Byrne, G. J . . Harnett, P. (2016). Mindfulness for motor and nonmotor dysfunctions in Parkinson's disease. *Parkinsons Disease*, Article ID 7109052.

Donnelly, K. Z., Linnea, K., Grant, D. A., & Lichtenstein, J. (2014). The feasibility and impact of a yoga pilot programme on the quality-of-life of adults with acquired brain injury. *Brain Injury*, *31*(2), 208–214.

Elliot, B. (2011). Arts-based and narrative inquiry in liminal experience reveal platforming as basic social psychological process. *The Arts in Psychotherapy*, *38*, 96–103.

Evans, J. J. (2011). Positive psychology and brain injury rehabilitation. *Brain Impairment*, *12*(2), 117–127.

Evans, J. J., & Cullen, B. (In Press). Positive psychotherapy for neurological conditions. In G. N. Yeates & F. Ashworth (Eds.), *Psychological therapies in neuropsychological rehabilitation*. Hove: Psychology Press.

Fisk, J. D., Ritvo, P. G., Ross, L., Haasem, D. A., Marrie, T. J., & Schlech, W. F. (1994). Measuring the functional impact of fatigue: Initial validation of the fatigure impact scale. *Clinical Infectious Disease*, *18*(Supplement 1), s79–83.

Fitzpatrick, L., Simpson, J., & Smith, A. (2010). A qualitative analysis of Mindfulness-Based Cognitive Therapy (MBCT) in Parkinson's disease. *Psychology & Psychotherapy*, *83*, 179–192.

Gao, Q., Leung, A., Yang, Y., Wei, Q., Guan, M., Jia, C., & He, C. (2014). Effects of Tai Chi on balance and fall prevention in Parkinson's disease: A randomized controlled trial. *Clinical Rehabilitation*, *28*, 748–753.

Gemmell, C., & Leathem, J. M. (2006). A study investigating the effects of tai chi chuan: Individuals with traumatic brain injury compared to controls. *Brain Injury*, *20*, 151–156.

Gracey, F., Ford, C., & Psaila, K. (2015). A provisional transdiagnostic cognitive behavioural model of post brain injury emotional adjustment. *NeuroDisability and Psychotherapy*, *3*, 154–185.

Grossman, P., Kappos, L., Gensicke, H., D'Souza, M., Mohr, D., Penner, I., & Steiner, C. (2010). MS quality of life, depression and fatigue improve after mindfulness training. *Neurology*, *75*, 1141–1149.

Hackney, M. E., & Earhart, G. M. (2008). Tai Chi improves balance and mobility in people with Parkinson disease. *Gait & Posture*, *28*, 456–460.

Haslam, C., Holme, A., Haslam, S. A., Lyer, A., Jetten, J., & Williams, W.H. (2008). Maintaining group memberships: Social identity continuity predicts well-being after stroke. *Neuropsychological Rehabilitation*, *18*, 671–691

Hart, J., Kanner, H., Gilboa-Mayo, R., Haroeh-Peer, O., Rozenthul-Sorokin, N., & Eldar, R. (2004). Tai Chi Chuan practice in community-dwelling persons after stroke. *International Journal of Rehabilitation Research*, *27*, 303–304.

Hilari, K., Needle, J. J., & Harrison, K. L. (2012). What are the important factors in health-related quality of life for people with aphasia? A systematic review. *Archives of Physical Medicine & Rehabilitation*, *93*(Supplement 1), 86–95.

Hoogerwerf, A. E. W., Bol, Y., Lobbestael, J., Hupperts, R., & van Heugten, C. M. (2017). Mindfulness-based cognitive therapy for severely fatigued multiple sclerosis patients: A waiting list controlled study. *Journal of Rehabilitation Medicine*, *49*(6), 497–504.

Hwang, I., Song, R., Ahn, S., Lee, M., Wayne, P., & Sohn, M. K. (2017). Exploring the adaptability of Tai Chi to stroke rehabilitation. *Rehabilitation Nursing*, Published Ahead of Print, 4th October.

Jacobson, N. S., & Truax, P. (1991). Clinical significance: A statistical approach to defining meaningful change in psychotherapy research. *Journal of Consulting and Clinical Psychology*, *59*, 12–19.

Jahnke, R., Larkey, L., Rogers, C., Etnier, J., & Lin, F. (2012). A comprehensive review of health benefits of qi gong and tai chi. *American Journal of Health Promotion, 24*(6), e1–e25.

Johansson, B., Bjhur, H., & Rönnbäck, L. (2012). Mindfulness-Based Stress Reduction (MBSR) improves long-term mental fatigue after stroke and traumatic brain injury. *Brain Injury, 26*, 1621–1628.

Kabat-Zinn, J. (2003). Mindfulness-based interventions in context: Past, present and future. *Clinical Psychology: Science & Practice, 10*, 144–156.

Kaplan-Solms, K., & Solms, M. (2000). *Clinical studies in neuro-psychoanalysis: An introduction to a depth neuropsychology*. London: Karnac.

Kaltenmark, M. (1969). *Lao Tzu and Taoism* (Roger Greaves, Trans.). Stanford, CA: Stanford University Press.

Kauhanen, M., Korpelainen, J. T., Hiltunen, P., Busin, E., Mononen, H., Maatta, R., . . . Myllyla, V. V. (1999). Poststroke depression correlates with cognitive impairment and neurological deficits. *Stroke, 30*(9), 1875–1880.

Kenuk, S., & Porter, H. (2017). The outcomes for mindfulness-based interventions for adults who have experienced a traumatic brain injury: A systematic review of the literature. *American Journal of Recreation Therapy, 16*(2).

Kolahkaj, B., & Zargar, F. (2015). Effect of mindfulness-based stress reduction on anxiety, depression and stress in women with multiple sclerosis. *Nursing and Midwifery Studies, 4*(4), e29655.

Kutlubaev, M. A., & Hackett, M. L. (2014). Predictors of depression after stroke and impact of depression on stroke outcome: An updated systematic review of observational studies. *International Journal of Stroke, 9*(8), 1026–1036.

Laures-Gore, J., & Shisler Marshall, R. (2016). Mindfulness meditation in aphasia: A case report. *NeuroRehabilitation, 38*, 321–329.

Lazaridou, A., Philbrook, P., & Tzika, A. A. (2013). Yoga and mindfulness as therapeutic interventions for stroke rehabilitation: A systematic review. *Evidence-based Complementary and Alternative Medicine: eCAM, 2013*, 357108.

Lee, B. (2000). *Striking thoughts: Bruce Lee's wisdom for daily living*. New York: Tuttle Publishing.

Li, F., Harmer, P., Fitzgerald, K. J., Eckstrom, E., Stock, R., Galver, J. . . . Batya, S. S. (2012). Tai Chi and postural stability in patients with Parkinson's disease. *New England Journal of Medicine, 366*, 511–519.

Little, J., & Lee, B. (2000). *Bruce Lee: A warrior's journey* (TV Documentary). Warner Home Video.

Lundgren, T., Dahl, J., Yardi, N., & Melin, L. (2008). Acceptance and commitment therapy and yoga for drug-refractory epilepsy: A randomized controlled trial. *Epilepsy & Behaviour, 13*(1), 102–108.

Lynton, H., Kligler, B., & Shiflett, S. (2007). Yoga in stroke rehabilitation: A systematic review and results of a pilot study. *Topics in Stroke Rehabilitation, 14*(4), 1–8.

Lyu, D., Lyu, X., Zhang, Y., Ren, Y., Yang, F., Zhou, L., Zou, Y., & Li, Z. (2018). Tai Chi for stroke rehabilitation: A systematic review and meta-analysis of randomized controlled trials. *Frontiers in Physiology, 9*, 983. https://doi.org/10.3389/fphys.2018.00983

Mańko, G., Ziółkowski, A., Mirski, A., & Kłosiński, M. (2013). The effectiveness of selected Tai Chi exercises in a program of strategic rehabilitation aimed at improving self-care skills of patients aroused from prolonged coma after severe TBI. *Medical*

Science Monitor: International Medical Journal of Experimental and Clinical Research, 19, 767–771.

Mazzarin, C. M., Valderramas, S. R., de Paula, F. M., Tiepolo, E., Guérios, L., Parisotto, D., & Israel, V. L. (2017). Effects of Dance and of Tai Chi on functional mobility, balance, and agility in Parkinson disease. *Topics in Geriatric Rehabilitation, 33*(4), 262–272.

McHugh, L., & Wood, R. (2013). Stimulus over-selectivity in temporal brain injury: Mindfulness as a potential intervention. *Brain Injury, 27*, 1595–1599.

McMillan, T., Robertson, I. H., Brock, D., & Chorlton, L. (2002). Brief mindfulness training for attentional problems after traumatic brain injury: A randomised control treatment trial. *Neuropsychological Rehabilitation, 12*, 117–125.

Menlove, L., Crayton, E., Kneebone, I., et al. (2015). Predictors of anxiety after stroke: A systematic review of observational studies. *Journal of Stroke & Cerebrovascular Disease, 24*, 107–1117.

Merton, T. (1969). *The way of Chuang Tzu*. New York: New Directions.

Mills, N., & Allen, J. (2000). Mindfulness of movement as a coping strategy in multiple sclerosis: A pilot study. *General Hospital Psychiatry, 22*(6), 425–431.

Moustgaard, A., Bedard, M., & Felteau, M. (2007). Mindfulness-Based Cognitive Therapy (MBCT) for individuals who had a stroke: Results from a Pilot 90 study. *The Journal of Cognitive Rehabilitation, 25*(4), 4–10.

Ni, X., Liu, S., Lu, F., Shi, X., & Guo, X. (2014, June 13). Efficacy and safety of Tai Chi for Parkinson's disease: A systematic review and meta-analysis of randomized controlled trials. *PLoS ONE*. https://doi.org/10.1371/journal.pone.0099377

Orenstein, E., Basilakos, A., & Shisler Marshall, R. (2012). Effects of mindfulness meditation on three individuals with aphasia. *International Journal of Language & Communication Disorders/Royal College of Speech & Language Therapists, 47*(6), 673–684. https://doi.org/10.1111/j.1460-6984.2012.00173.x

Parr, S. (2001). Psychosocial aspects of aphasia: Whose perspectives? *Folia Phoniatrica & Logopaedica, 53*, 266–288.

Pickut, B. A., Van Hecke, W., Kerckhofs, E., Mariën, P., Vanneste, S., Cras, P., & Parizel, P. M. (2013). Mindfulness based intervention in Parkinson's disease leads to structural brain changes on MRI: A randomized controlled longitudinal trial. *Clinical Neurology & Neurosurgery, 115*(12), 2419–2425.

Pickut, B. A., Vanneste, S., Hirsch, M. A., Van Hecke, W., Kerckhofs, E., Marien, P. . . . Cras, P. (2015). Mindfulness training among individuals with Parkinson's disease: Neurobehavioral effects. *Parkinson's Disease*, Article ID 816404.

Quinn, D., & Jones, K. (2012). Tai Chi Movement (TMW) and embodied mindfulness in mental and physical health. *Inservice Presentation for Herefordshire Primary Care Trust*, UK.

Radder, D. L., Sturkenboom, I. H., van Nimwegen, M., Keus, S. H., Bloem, B. R., & de Vries, N. M. (2017). Physical therapy and occupational therapy in Parkinson's disease. *International Journal of Neuroscience*, 1–14.

Rajesh, B., Jayachandran, D., Mohandas, G., & Radhakrishnan, K. (2006). A pilot study of a yoga meditation protocol for patients with medically refractory epilepsy. *The Journal of Alternative and Complementary Medicine, 12*(4), 367–371.

Rivkin, N. (2013). *The effect of yoga on aphasia rehabilitation*. Unpublished Thesis. Appalachian State University, Boone, NC.

Roland, K. P. (2014). Applications of yoga in Parkinson's disease: A systematic literature review. *Journal of Parkinsonism & Restless Legs Syndrome, 4*, 1–8.

Ross, K., Howe, T., Jenstad, L., & Sinden, E. (2018). Developing a communicatively-accessible group yoga class for adults with aphasia post-stroke. *Aphasiology*, *32*(Supplement 1), 189–190.

Russell, T. A. (2011). Body in mind training: Mindful movement for severe and enduring mental illness. *British Journal of Wellbeing*, *2*(4), 13–16.

Russell, T. A., & Tatton-Ramos, T. (2014). Body in mind training: Mindful movement for the clinical setting. *Neuro-Disability & Psychotherapy*, *2*(1/2), 108–136.

Sather, T. W. (2015). *Flow experiences amongst individuals with Aphasia*. Ph.D. Dissertations, Western Michigan University, 1196.

Schaffer, O. (2013). *Crafting fun user experiences: A method to facilitate flow*. Fairfield, IA: Human Factors International.

Schmid, A. A., Miller, K. K., Van Puymbroeck, M., & Schalk, N. (2016). Feasibility and results of a case study of yoga to improve physical functioning in people with chronic traumatic brain injury. *Disability & Rehabilitation*, *38*(9), 914–920.

Senders, A., Bourdette, D., Hanes, D., Vijaysgree, Y., & Shinto, L. (2014). Perceived stress in multiple sclerosis the potential role of mindfulness in health and well-being. *Journal of Evidence-Based Complementary & Alternative Medicine*, *19*(2), 104–111.

Shadden, B. B. (2005). Aphasia as identity theft (theory and practice). *Aphasiology*, *19*, 211–223.

Shapira, M. Y., Chelouche, M., Yanai, R., Kaner, C., & Szold, A. (2001). Tai Chi Chuan practice as a tool for rehabilitation of severe head trauma: 3 case reports. *Archives of Physical Medicine & Rehabilitation*, *82*(9), 1283–1285.

Shisler-Marshall, R., Lores-Gore, J., & Love, K. (2017). Brief mindfulness meditation group training in aphasia: Exploring attention, language and psychophysiological outcomes. *International Journal of Language & Communication Disorders*, *53*(1), 40–54.

Shravat, A. (2014). The role of a Yoga group within a holistic rehabilitation setting for ABI using compassion focused therapy approach. A qualitative case illustration. *Neuro-Disability & Psychotherapy*, *2*(1/2), 100–107.

Silverthorne, C., Khalsa, S. B., Gueth, R., DeAvilla, N., & Pansini, J. (2012). Respiratory, physical, and psychological benefits of breath-focused yoga for adults with severe Traumatic Brain Injury (TBI): A brief pilot study report. *International Journal of Yoga Therapy*, *22*(1), 47–51.

Simpson, R., Booth, J., Lawrence, M., Byrne, S., Mair, F., & Mercer, S. (2014). Mindfulness 21 based interventions in multiple sclerosis: A systematic review. *BMC Neurology*, *14*(22), 15.

Simpson, R., Byrne, S., Wood, K., Mair, F. S., & Mercer, S. W. (2018). *Optimising mindfulness-based stress reduction for people with multiple sclerosis*. London: Sage Publications.

Simpson, R., Mair, F. S., & Mercer, S. W. (2017). Mindfulness-based stress reduction for people with multiple sclerosis: A feasibility randomised controlled trial. *BMC Neurology*, *17*(1), 141.

Sungkarat, S., Boripuntakul, S., Chattipakorn, N., Watcharasaksilp, K., & Lord, S. R. (2017). Effects of tai chi on cognition and fall risk in older adults with mild cognitive impairment: A randomized controlled trial. *Journal of the American Geriatrics Society*, *65*, 721–727.

Tang, V., Poon, W. S., & Kwan, P. (2015). Mindfulness-based therapy for drug-resistant epilepsy: An assessor-blinded randomized trial. *Neurology*, *85*(13), 1100–1107.

Tavee, J., Rensel, M., Planchon, S. M., Butler, R. S., & Stone, L. (2011). Effects of meditation on pain and quality of life in multiple sclerosis and peripheral neuropathy. *International Journal of MS Care, 13*, 163–168.

Taylor-Piliae, R. E., Hoke, T. M., Hepworth, J. T., Latt, L. D., Najafi, B. . . .Coull, B. M. (2014). Effect of Tai Chi on physical function, fall rates and quality of life among older stroke survivors. *Archives of Physical Medicine and Rehabilitation, 95*, 816–824.

Thompson, N. J., Patel, A. H., Selwa, L. M., Stoll, S. C., Begley, C. E., Johnson, E. K. . . . Fraser, R. T. (2015). Expanding the efficacy of project UPLIFT: Distance delivery of mindfulness-based depression prevention to people with epilepsy. *Journal of Consulting and Clinical Psychology, 83*(2), 304–313.

Todd, D., & Smith, M. (In Press). Acceptance and commitment therapy. In G. N. Yeates & F. Ashworth (Eds.), *Psychological therapies in neuropsychological rehabilitation*. Hove: Psychology Press.

Toh, S. F. M. (2013). A systematic review on the effectiveness of Tai Chi exercise in individuals with Parkinson's disease from 2003 to 2013. *Hong Kong Journal of Occupational Therapy, 23*, 69–81.

Tyerman, A., & Humphrey, M. (1984). Changes in self concept following severe head injury. *International Journal of Rehabilitation Research, 7*, 11–23.

Vergara-Diaz, G., Osypiuk, K., Hausdorff, J. M., Bonato, P., Gow, B. J., Miranda, J. G., et al. (2018). Tai Chi for reducing dual-task gait variability, a potential mediator of fall risk in Parkinson's disease: A pilot randomized controlled trial. *Global Advances in Health & Medicine, 7*, 216495611877538

Wang, C., Bannuru, R., Ramel, J., Kupelnick, B., Scott, T., & Schmid, C. H. (2010). Tai Chi on psychological well-being: Systematic review and meta-analysis. *BMC Complementary Alternative Medicine, 10*, 23.

Whiting, D., Simpson, G., Ciarrochi, J., & McLeod, H. (2012). Assessing the feasibility pf Acceptance and Commitment Therapy in promoting psychological adjustment after severe traumatic brain injury. *Brain Injury, 26*(4–5), 588–589.

Winser, S. J., Kannan, P., Pang, M., Smith, C., & Tsang, W. W. (2018). Potential benefits and safety of T'ai Chi for balance and functional independence in people with cerebellar ataxia. *The Journal of Alternative and Complimentary Medicine, 24*(12), 1221–1223.

Winser, S. J., Kannan, P., Pang, M., & Tsang, W. W. (2017). Tai chi for improving balance in cerebellar ataxia: A feasibility. *Archives of Physical Medicine & Rehabilitation, 98*(10), e113–e114.

Winser, S. J., Tsang, W. W., Krishnamurthy, K., & Kannan, P. (2018). Does Tai Chi improve balance and reduce falls incidence in neurological disorders? A systematic review and meta-analysis. *Clinical Rehabilitation, 32*(9), 1157–1168.

Wu, S., Chen, J., Wang, S., Jiang, M., Wang, X., & Wen, Y. (2018). Effect of Tai Chi exercise on balance function of stroke patients: A meta-analysis. *Medical Science Monitor Basic Research, 24*, 210–215.

Xie, G. L., Rao, T., Lin, L., Lin, Z., Xiao, T., Yang, M. . . . Chen, L. (2018). Effects of Tai Chi Yunshou exercise on community-based stroke patients: A cluster randomized controlled trial. *European Review of Aging and Physical Activity, 15*, 17.

Yang, Y., Li, X.-Y., Gong, L., Zhu, Y.-L., & Hao, Y.-L. (2014). Tai Chi for improvement of motor function, balance and gait in Parkinson's disease: A systematic review and meta-analysis. *PLoS ONE, 9*(7), Article ID e102942.

Yan Li, G., Wang, W., Liu, G. L., & Zhang, Y. (2018). Effects of Tai Chi on balance and gait in stroke survivors: A systematic meta-analysis of randomized controlled trials. *Journal of Rehabilitation Medicine*, *50*(7), 582–588.

Yeates, G. N. (2014). Using pagers and alerts as adjuncts to psychological therapies following acquired brain injury. In A. Cantagallo (Ed.), *Telerehabilitation and Adaptations: Assistive Technology for People with Neuropsychological Impairments*. Milan: FrancoAngeli.

Yeates, G. N. (2015). Flow state experiences as a biopsychosocial guide for Tai Ji intervention and research in neuro-rehabilitation. *Neuro-Disability & Psychotherapy*, *3*(1).

Yeates, G. N. (2018). Flow state experiences as a biopsychosocial guide for Tai Ji intervention and research in neuro-rehabilitation. In G. N. Yeates & G. Farrell (Eds.), *Neuro-disability & psychotherapy, specialist topics (Vol. I): Eastern influences on neuropsychotherapy: Accepting, soothing and stilling cluttered and critical minds in neurological conditions*. Oxford: Routledge.

Yeates, G. N. (2019). Eastern spirituality, mind-body practices and neuro-rehabilitation. In A. Coles & J. Collicutt (Eds.), *The neurology of religion* (pp. 191–213). Cambridge: Cambridge University Press.

Yeates, G. N. (in press). The potential contribution of mind-body interventions within psychological support following aphasia: A conceptual review and case study. In G. N. Yeates & K. Meredith (Eds.), *Neuro-disability & psychotherapy, specialist topics (volume II). Psychotherapy & aphasia: Supporting emotions & relationships*. Oxford: Routledge.

Yeates, G. N., & Farrell, G. (2014). Editorial for special issue: "Accepting, soothing and stilling cluttered and critical minds in neurological conditions: The influence of Eastern practices". *Neuro-Disability & Psychotherapy*, *2*(1/2), 1–2.

Yeates, G. N., & Farrell, G. (2018). Editors' forward. In G. N. Yeates & G. Farrell (Eds.), *Neuro-disability & psychotherapy, specialist topics (Vol. I): Eastern influences on neuropsychotherapy: Accepting, soothing and stilling cluttered and critical minds in neurological conditions*. Oxford: Routledge.

Yeates, G. N., Hamill, M., Sutton, L., Psaila, K., Mohamed, S., & O'Dell, J. (2008). Dysexecutive problems and interpersonal relating following frontal brain injury: reformulation in cognitive-analytic therapy. *Neuropsychoanalysis, 10*, 43–58.

Yeates, G. N., Murphy, M., Baldwin, J., Wilkes, J., & Mahadevan, M. (2015). A pilot evaluation of a yoga group for survivors of acquired brain injury in a community setting. *Clinical Psychology Forum, 267*, 46–51.

Yeates, G. N., Nagrani, S., Smith, A., Dorney-Savage, J., Whitman, J., & Khan. E. (submitted). Diversity of needs in tai chi (taiji) group interventions following acquired brain injury: A mixed methods study.

Zhang, L., Layne, C., Lowder, T., & Liu, J. (2011). A review focused on the psychological effectiveness of Tai Chi on different populations. *Evidence-based Complementary & Alternative Medicine*, 1–9.

Zheng, G., Zhou, W., Xia, R., Tao, J., & Chen, L. (2016). Aerobic exercises for cognition rehabilitation following stroke: A systematic review. *Journal of Stroke and Cerebrovascular Diseases*, *25*, 2780–2789. https://doi.org/10.1016/j.jstrokecerebrovasdis.2016.07.035

Zhou, J., Yin, T., Gao, Q., & Yang, X. C. (2015). A meta-analysis on the efficacy of Tai Chi in patients with Parkinson's disease between 2008 and 2014. *Evidence Based Complementary and Alternative Medicine*, *2015*, 593263.

Zigmond, A. S., & Snaith, R. P. (1983). The hospital anxiety and depression scale. *Acta Psychiatrica Scandinavica, 67*(6), 361–370. https://doi.org/10.1111/j.1600-0447.1983.tb09716.x

Zou, L., Wang, C., Chen, X., & Wang, H. (2018). Baduanjin exercise for stroke rehabilitation: A systematic review with meta-analysis of randomized controlled trials. *International Journal of Environmental Research & Public Health, 15*, 600.

Zou, L., Yeung, A., Zeng, N., Wang, C., Sun, L., Thomas, G., & Wang, H. (2018). Effects of mind-body exercises for mood and functional capabilities in post-stroke patients: An analytical review of randomized controlled trials. *International Journal of Environmental Research & Public Health, 15*, 721.

Index

Note: Page numbers in italics indicate figures and page numbers in bold indicate tables.

Aachner Aphasie Test (AAT) 86
acceptance and commitment therapy (ACT) 23–24, 138–139
acoustico-mnestic aphasia 18, 20, 29
acquired brain injury (ABI): aphasia and 53–54, 72, 80; children and 95–96, 98; emotional support and 137; family relationships and 53–56, 66, 74; family therapists and 54; healthcare externalisation and 65; impact on self-identity 55; neurological rehabilitation and 81, 136–137; psychotherapy and 137; speech and language therapists (SLTs) and 55; tai ji and 142–143, 149–151
Ahn, S. 142–143
Allen, J. 142
amnestic aphasia 18
Anti-Anorexia league 65
aphasia: acoustico-mnestic 18, 20, 29; acquired brain injury (ABI) and 53–54, 72, 80; amnestic 18; as horizontal stressor 57; impact of 33; parents with 72–73; psychoeducation and 6; receptive 17, 20, 25–26; semantic 18, 21, 25, 29, 31; social approach to 80–82; social construction impacts 61; social model of 55; story-telling and 62; stroke and 1, 80; *see also* people with aphasia
Aphasia Action Success and Knowledge (ASK) therapy 7
aphasia rehabilitation: family therapists and 54, 68; group aphasia therapy and 80, 82–83; interventions for 6–8; narrative therapy and 64–65; psychotherapy approach to 83; social approach and 81–82; social constructionism and 64–65; Talking Mats approach 55; Total Communication strategies 55; *see also* neurological rehabilitation; personal construct psychology (PCP)
asana yoga 139
ASHA NOMS 86
Asian spiritual traditions 138, 144–146
Assessment for Living with Aphasia (ALA) 6
Association for Family Therapy and Systemic Practice (AFT) 56
auditory-verbal information 23, 25–29
Australia 1
Azizi, H. 140

Baker, C. 6, 8
Bannuru, R. 141
Basilakos, A. 108, 144
Batson, M. 142
Beck Depression Inventory (BDI) 86, 118
Bedard, M. 139
Behavioural Outcomes of Anxiety (BOA) scale 5
belongingness 89–90
Bion, W. R. 88
Birmingham Cognitive Screen (BCoS) 23, 25, 28
Bishop, D. V. 19
Bishop, S. R. 108
Blackman, N. M. D. 83
Blake, H. 142
Brady, M. C. 2
Brumfitt, S. 51, 83
Buddhism 138

Burschka, J. M. 142–143
Butler, R. S. 142
Byng, S. 33

Caplan, D. 17
Caregiver Burden Inventory (CBI) 86
caregivers 81, 83, **86**, 91; *see also* family relationships
case studies: AF (mindfulness intervention) 122, *123–124*; Andy (tai ji group) 151–152, **152–153**, 154, **154**, 155; Barry and Kay (SLT and family therapy) 69–72; Ben (stepped care) 8–9, **9–10**; Cathy and Ruth (personal construct psychology) 36–51; CF (mindfulness intervention) 124, *125*, 126, *126*; GM (mindfulness intervention) 126–127, *128*, 129, *129*; MB (mindfulness intervention) 119–120, *120–121*, 122; Ms. A (semantic aphasia intervention) 21–29; Rose (mindfulness intervention) 109–113; Theo (structured narrative therapy) 99–102, **103**, 104, **104**, 105
Centro Afasia CIRP: assessment of needs and 84; bio-psycho-social perspective in 113; Conversazione Narrativa workshop 84–89; group analysis approach and 80; group aphasia therapy and 80, 83; integrated theatre group and 83; mindfulness interventions and 114–118
Chan Buddhism 145
Chelouche, M. 142
Chen, J. 141
Chen, L. 141
Chen, X. 141
child development 95–96, 98
children: acquired brain injury (ABI) and 95–96, 98; family therapy and 72–73; narrative intervention for 95–96; parental roles and 73
Children's Trust 95
circumspection 44
cognitive behavioural therapy (CBT) 23, 65, 137
communication disorders: couple relationships and 67, 69–72; family relationships and 58–61; family therapists and 68; healthcare externalisation and 65; impact on psychotherapy 137; mindfulness interventions and 138; story-telling and 62; *see also* aphasia
comprehension training 20
Confucionism 145
constructive alternativism 33–34
control 44
Conversazione Narrativa workshop: Centro Afasia CIRP and 84–85; evaluation measures 86–87; evaluation of change and retest 89; goals of 84; group intervention 87–91; individual phase 85–87; methods 85; psychotherapists and 88; speech and language therapists (SLTs) and 88; supportive conversation techniques 88
Corriveau, H. 142
Coull, B. M. 141
countertransference 20–21, 24, 28
couple relationships 53, 67, 69–72, 83
CPC cycle (circumspection, pre-emption, control) 44–46, 50
Cramer, H. 140
Create Integration Resiliency Possibility (CIRP) – Aphasia Center of Turin *see* Centro Afasia CIRP
Crielesi, M. 109, 144
Crowe, S. 66
Csíkszentmihályi, M. 147

Dalton, P. 34–36
Dao De Ching 146
Daoism 140, 144–149
DeAvilla, N. 139
Defloor, T. 53
Desrochers, P. 142
Dickinson, J. 108, 144
Ding, M. 141
Dobos, G. 140
Donnelly, K. Z. 139
Dorney-Savage, J. 143

ecomaps 57, 60, *60*
emotional adjustment 17–19, 137–139
epilepsy 139

family identity 55
family life cycle 57–58, *58*, *59*
family relationships: acquired brain injury (ABI) and 53–56, 74; communication disorders and 58–61; coping mechanisms in 66–68; ecomaps 60, *60*; people with aphasia and 64–66, 68–69, 72; rehabilitation professionals and 74–75; resilience and 65–68, 75; stress and 53, 57

family therapy: acquired brain injury (ABI) rehabilitation and 54; aphasia rehabilitation and 54, 68; children and 72–73; communication disorders and 68; defining 56; genograms and 58; mental health services and 56; neuro-rehabilitation training in 54, 73–74; speech and language therapists (SLTs) and 54, 68, 70–71
Farrell, G. 139
Felteau, M. 139
Five Element Theory (Wuxing) 146
Five Facet Mindfulness Questionnaire (FFMQ) 118, 130
flow psychology 146–148
Flow States 147–151
Fransella, F. 35
Fredrick, A. 2
Freud, S. 17
Friary, P. 108, 144
Functional Assessment of Communication Skills for Adults (I-ASHA-FACS) 86

Gailey, G. 83
Gao, Q. 141
Gemmell, C. 142
genograms 57–59, *59*, 67
Gilpin, S. 33
Goal Attainment Scaling (GAS) 100–102
Grant, D. A. 139
group analysis approach 80
group aphasia therapy: aphasia rehabilitation and 80, 82–83; contribution of caregiver 91; Conversazione Narrativa workshop 84–91; efficacy of 82, 90–91; integrated theatre group 83; mindfulness and 113–119, 129–130
Grypdonck, M. 53
Guan, M. 141
Gueth, R. 139

He, C. 141
healthcare externalisation 65
Hepworth, J. T. 141
Hildebrandt, N. 17
Hoke, T. M. 141
Horan, J. J. 20
Hospital Anxiety and Depression Scale (HADS) 5, 152
Hudson, K. 6, 8
Hwang, I. 142–143

impairment-focused therapy 82
intensive short-term dynamic psychotherapy (ISTDP) 24
Ireland, C. 33

Jia, C. 141
Jiang, M. 141
Jones, K. 143

Kagan, A. 82
Kairy, D. 142
Kaner, C. 142
Kannan, P. 141–142
Kaplan-Solms, K. 17–18, 25
Kelly, G. 33–35
Keune, P. M. 142–143
Khalsa, S. B. 139
Khan, E. 143
Kinsella, G. 66
Kłosiński, M. 142
Kneebone, I. I. 1, 4, 5, 9
Krishnamurthy, K. 141
Kuhn, P. 142–143
Kupelnick, B. 141

lacunar stroke 21
Langhorst, J. 140
language: deficits in 18, 20; emotional adjustment and 17; narrative therapy and 84–86; receptive 21; receptive deficits 20, 28–29, 56–57; recovery of 1; rehabilitation interventions for 82–83; social power and 62–64; social relationships and 33, 61; syntax and 18, 20–21; Total Communication strategies and 57; *see also* aphasia; communication disorders
Lao Tzu 146
Latt, L. D. 141
Lauche, R. 140
Laures-Gore, J. 108, 144
Leathem, J. M. 142
Lee, B. 148
Lee, M. 142–143
Leung, A. 141
Lewis, L. 20, 28
Li, Z. 141
Lichtenstein, J. 139
Life Participation Approach to Aphasia (LPAA) 81, 113–115
liminality 148–149
Lin, L. 141

Lin, Z. 141
Lincoln, N. 1
Linnea, K. 139
Liu, G. L. 141
Luria, A. R. 18, 21, 25, 28–29
Lykke Mortensen, E. 53
Lyu, D. 141
Lyu, X. 141

Magdalene Sisters, The 22
Mańko, G. 142
Marshall, J. C. 17
Marshall, R. S. 108, 144
McCann, C. M. 108, 144
meaning-making 17–21, 28
meditation 116, 139–140, 144; *see also* mindfulness interventions
mental health 1–2
mental health services 2–3, 23–24, 56
Miller, K. K. 139
Mills, N. 142
mind-body interventions: Asian spiritual traditions 138; Daoist frameworks for 144–146; emotional support and 137; flow psychology and 146–148; liminality and 148–149; mindfulness and 138–139; neurological rehabilitation and 138–149, 155; people with aphasia and 143–144; tai ji and 138, 140–143, 149–155; yoga and 138–140
Mindfulness-Based Cognitive Therapy (MBCT) 115
mindfulness interventions: anxiety reduction and 109; assessments for 118; case studies in 119–120, *120*, 121, *121*, 122, *123*, 124, *124–125*, 126, *126*, 127, *128*, 129, *129*; detailed case study formulation *111*; divided attention and 108; emotional support and 138; group evaluations 113–119, 129–130; individual sessions and 109–113; mind-body interventions and 138–139; neurological rehabilitation and 138–139; Parkinson's disease and 138; participants in **116**; people with aphasia and 108–131, 144; results of **118–119**
Mirski, A. 142
Modified Fatigue Impact Scale (M-FIS) 152
Monopoli, G. 109, 144
Monte, S. 144
mood disorders 5–6, **9–10**
mood problems: case study formulations and *111*; family therapy for 75; mind-body interventions for 140–142; mindfulness interventions and 130; people with aphasia and 5–6, 8, 23, 28, 31, 109–110, 112–113; post-stroke 2; screening for 5–6, **86**, 118
Moustgaard, A. 139
multiple sclerosis 140, 142
'My Beautiful Broken Brain' 49

Nagrani, S. 143
Najafi, B. 141
narrative therapy 61–62, 64; *see also* structured narrative therapy (SNT)
Neidan process 145
neurological damage 17, 20, 35
neurological rehabilitation: acoustico-mnestic aphasia and 18; acquired brain injury (ABI) and 81, 136–137; aims of 81; emotional influences on 136–137; family relationships and 74–75; family therapy training and 54, 73–74; linguistic limitations in 136; mind-body interventions for 137–149, 155; mindfulness interventions and 138–139; normal mourning in 20; physiotherapy interventions and 136–137; poetry and 18, 26–27; professional limitations in 136–137; syntax in 20–21; systemic formulation in 74–75; tai ji and 138, 140–143, 149–151; writing and 18, 26, 29; yoga and 139–140; *see also* aphasia rehabilitation
neuropsychological assessment 20–21, 24, 28
normal mourning 17–20, 26–28
Norup, A. 53

O'Byrne, L. 6, 8
Orenstein, E. 108, 144
Oschman, P. 142–143
Oy, Y. 142–143

Paediatric Neurocognitive Intervention (PNI) 96, 98
Pan, S. 142
Pang, M. 142
Pansini, J. 139
Parkinson's disease 138, 140–141, 143
Parr, S. 33
Patterson, K. 19

people with aphasia: assessment of needs and 84; belongingness 89–90; changes in identity and 107–108; children and 72–73; communication support tools for 8; contribution of caregiver 91; couple relationships and 53, 83; family communication strategies 68–69; family relationships and 64–66, 72; flow states in 151; group intervention and 87–91, 113–130; impact of disrespect on 62–63, *63*, 64, 75; mental health and 1–2; mental health services and 2–3; mind-body interventions for 143–144; mindfulness and 108–131, 144; personal construct psychology (PCP) and 33, 36–51; screening for mood problems 5–6, **86**, 118; service provision to 2; social participation by 82–83; stepped psychological care and 5–8, 10–11; stroke rehabilitation interventions for 6–8; suicide risk 8; syntax assessments 19; yoga and 144; *see also* aphasia; aphasia rehabilitation
perforated consciousness 18
Perlesz, A. 66
personal construct psychology (PCP): case studies in 36–51; constructive alternativism in 33–34; counselling in 35–36; CPC cycle in 44–46, 50; 'credulous' listening approach in 50–51; neurological rehabilitation and 35; people with aphasia and 33, 36–51; person as scientist in 33–34; professional constructs in 35; reflexivity in 33–35; stammering and 35; Talking Mats approach 48, *48*, 49; two 'experts' in 50; value of creativity in 50
person as scientist 33–34
physiotherapy interventions 136–137
Planchon, S. M. 142
poetry 18, 26–27
positive stories (PS) of identity 101, **101**, 102
'Possibilities are Endless, The' 49
pre-emption 44
psychodynamic therapy 137
psychoeducation 6
Psycholinguistic Assessments of Language Assessments in Aphasia (PALPA) 19
psychotherapy: countertransference in 29; flow states in 147; identity and 149; intensive short-term dynamic 24; mindfulness and 138–139; reflexive consciousness and 18; rehabilitation and 81–83, 107–108; *see also* family therapy; group aphasia therapy; personal construct psychology (PCP)
Pyramids and Palm Trees Test 19

qi gong 145
Quality of Life after Brain Injury Inventory (QOLiBRI) 152
Quinn, D. 143

'Race For Life' campaign 65
Raja yoga 147
Ramel, J. 141
Rao, T. 141
receptive aphasia 17, 20, 25–26, 28–29, 31
receptive language deficits 28–29, 56–57
reflexive consciousness 18, 20, 31
reflexivity 33–35
Ren, Y. 141
Rensel, M. 142
resilience 65–68, 75
resilient therapy 66
Roche, L. 109
Roland, K. P. 140
Rose, M. 6, 8
Russell, T. A. 140
Ryan, B. 6, 8

Samyama 147
Sather, T. W. 151
Savage, M. C. 82
Schalk, N. 139
Schmid, A. A. 139
Schmid, C. H. 141
Scott, T. 141
self-identity 55
semantic aphasia 18, 25, 28–29, 31
semantics 17
Shapira, M. Y. 142
Shewell, C. 19
Shisler Marshall, R. 108, 144
Shravat, A. 139
Siert, L. 53
Signs of Depression Scale (SOD) 5
Silverthorne, C. 139
Simmons-Mackie, N. 82
single-word processing 19, *19*, 29, *30*
Smith, A. 143
Smith, C. 142

social approach 20, 80–82
social construction 61–62, 64–65
social model of aphasia 55
Sohn, M. K. 142–143
Solms, M. 17–18, 25
Song, R. 142–143
speech and language therapists (SLTs): acquired brain injury (ABI) and 55; family therapy and 54, 68, 70–71; mental health interventions by 3, 6; people with aphasia and 19; psychoeducation and 6; reflexive consciousness deficits and 20; stepped psychological care and 5–8, 11–12
speech pathologists *see* speech and language therapists (SLTs)
stammering 35
State-Trait Anxiety Inventory (STAIX) 118
stepped psychological care: case studies in 8–10; levels of intervention in 4, *4*, 5; people with aphasia and 5–8, 10–11; post-stroke access to 3–4, 10; speech pathologists and 5–8, 11–12
Stiell, K. 83
stimulation training 20
Stone, L. 142
story-telling 62
Stratton, P. 56
stress 53, 57
stroke 1, 6–8, 21, 80, 141–143
Stroke and Aphasia Quality of Life Scale (SAQoL-39) 6
Stroke Aphasic Depression Questionnaire-10 (SADQ-10) 5, 86, 118
Stroke Foundation (Australia) 2
Stroke Specific Quality of Life scale 130
structured narrative therapy (SNT): adult/child tensions in 104–105; aims of 98–99; autobiographical documents and 96, 100–101, 104; case studies in 99–105; developmental framework in 96, *97*, 98; Goal Attainment Scaling (GAS) in 100–102; interventions with 99–102, 104–105; positive stories (PS) of identity in 101, **101**, 102; practical application of 95–96; ratings of therapy outcome **103–104**; rationale for using 96, 98; summary of therapy sessions **102–103**
Sufi Dervishes 147
suicide risk 8
Supported Conversation for Adults with Aphasia (SCA) 81–82, 115
supportive conversation techniques 88
syntax: assessments considering 19, 31; comprehension and 17; deficits in 18, 25–26; emotional adjustment and 18–19; meaning-making and 17–21; receptive aphasia and 28–29, 31; reflexive consciousness and 18; semantic aphasia and 20–21
systemic formulation 74–75
systemic therapy 137
Szold, A. 142

tai ji: acquired brain injury (ABI) and 142–143, 149–151; adaptations for post-stroke difficulties **150–151**; case studies in 151–152, **152–153**, 154, **154**, 155; Daoist frameworks for 144–145; flow states in 148–151, 155; multiple sclerosis and 142; neurological rehabilitation and 138, 140–143, 149–151; Parkinson's disease and 141, 143; stroke rehabilitation and 141–143; traumatic brain injury (TBI) and 142
taijiquan 144
talking cure 18
Talking Mats approach 48, *48*, 49, 55
talking therapy 137–138
Tao, J. 141
Tavee, J. 142
Taylor-Piliae, R. E. 141
Teatro Babel 83
Test for the Reception of Grammar (TROG) 19
Test of Attention Matrices (TMA) 118
theatre groups 83
Total Communication strategies 55
Tousignant, M. 142
Trail Making Test (TMT) 118
traumatic brain injury (TBI) 53, 80, 136, 138–139, 142; *see also* acquired brain injury (ABI)
Tsang, W. W. 141–142

United Kingdom 53

Van Puymbroeck, M. 139
Verhaeghe, S. 53
Visual Analogue Mood Scales (VAMS) 86

Wang, C. 141
Wang, H. 141
Wang, S. 141
Wang, W. 141

Wang, X. 141
Wayne, P. 142–143
Wei, Q. 141
Wen, Y. 141
White, M. 95
Whitman, J. 143
Williams, B. 2
Winser, S. J. 141–142
World Health Organization (WHO) 81
Worrall, L. 6, 8, 82
writing 18, 26, 29
Wu S. 141
Wu Wei 146

Xia, R. 141
Xiao, T. 141
Xie, G. L. 141

Yanai, R. 142
Yang, F. 141
Yang, M. 141
Yang, Y. 141
Yan Li, G. 141
Yeates, G. N. 139, 143–144
yoga 138–140, 144, 147

Zhang, Y. 141
Zheng, G. 141
Zhou, L. 141
Zhou, W. 141
Zhuangzi 146
Ziółkowski, A. 142
Zou, L. 141
Zou, Y. 141